Born To Be Fit

Discover Your Natural Ability to Be
Healthy, Happy, and Fit.

Marguerite Brown, R.N.

Lockport NY Toronto Ontario

Tell Publishing
Published simultaneously in Lockport NY Toronto Ontario.

U.S.A.
5679 South Transit Rd. #181
Lockport NY 14094 U.S.A.
Tel. 1-800-726-8932

Canada
30 Kippendavie Avenue Toronto, Ontario
M4L 3R4 Canada
Tel. 1-800-726-8932

ISBN 1-896560-00-8
LCCN 95-061074
CIP C95-932033-4

Printed in the United States of America

*This book is dedicated to Peter and Nadia
whom I love very much.*

I sincerely thank Peter Brown, Nadia Heyd, Darrick Heyd, and Todd O'Connor for giving me their time without reservation, and who have encourgaed me, reviewed, and discussed with me many of the topics of this book that pertain to their fields of expertise.

Born To Be Fit

Table of Contents

Introduction

The human body is magnificent. It has mechanisms with incomprehensible sophistication which developed and prevailed throughout evolutionary history. We are very limited in understanding many of the body's complex physiological processes. The metabolic activities of the body are totally internal physiological functions aimed at sustaining life and well-being, and we have no control over these functions. Why do many of us think we can force our bodies to burn fat by rationing our dietary intake?

This book is an effort to explain that the body possess a tenacity and "wisdom" designed to preserve and sustain life and well-being *automatically*. The consumption and the use of energy by our bodies are not a simple balancing of energy intake to energy output, but rather are complex processes aimed at sustaining life and the well-being of the body as a whole. Therefore, our attempts to consciously regulate our energy intake to energy output to maintain a desired weight often do not work and disrupt many of our innate body processes.

Our bodies are designed with mechanisms which release neurochemicals and endorphins that will make us experience pleasure whenever we indulge ourselves in activities that promote our health and well-being.

By responding to our pleasure-seeking instincts we are compelled to do what we should do to make us healthy and fit. There is no need to attempt to manipulate our natural mechanisms that control all aspects of our health and well-being. We must respond to our bodies' natural design and find pleasure in all the activities that we do. By aiming to find satisfaction, contentment, and joy in everything that we do and think about, and by doing that which makes us feel good, we will meet all our physical and emotional needs, which also include our nutritional needs, and we will live long, prosperous, happy, and healthy lives. A slim, trim figure will be a spin-off benefit of a healthy lifestyle.

Marguerite Brown

Chapter 1

Insights Into Losing Weight

What Does It Mean To Be Healthy and Fit?

Many people view health and fitness in terms of having a specific physical dimension and weight. However, health, fitness and attractiveness cannot be measured by a weighing scale. While there are measurements that can be made to determine levels of health and fitness, health and fitness can be best described as a sensation. It is a joyous sensation, a positive lively energy that we feel when we are healthy. People who are healthy and fit are also vibrantly beautiful.

The idea that attractiveness has set specifications, and dimensions is misguided! To think that we can control our body weight and size by reducing our food intake to force our bodies to burn fat is also misguided! On the contrary, depriving ourselves of the foods that our bodies need can lead to metabolic weight disturbances which render us susceptible to becoming fat and chronically overweight in the long run.

Many people have the potential to develop their figures to an *even more* attractive shape than the slim, trim figure they are attempting to achieve. It is *how* they go about achieving a model figure which actually sabotages and prevents them from achieving their potential fitness levels and body shape and tone.

Being healthy and fit is an ongoing state of physical, emotional, and social well-being. It is the outcome of our participation in the activities that enhance our living experience. It means that all our body mechanisms are functioning at optimum capacity, allowing us to enjoy our lives and stay healthy. Our body mechanisms are designed to function *automatically* thus ensuring our health, fitness, and well-being.

When our bodies are functioning at optimum level, we have a healthy clear complexion, twinkling eyes, shining hair, and strong teeth. We are full of energy, we feel good about ourselves, our muscles develop to their maximum strength and size, and our metabolism rises. Every action and reaction of our body comes into play to deliver the most enjoyable and rewarding life we could ever imagine.

All our body mechanisms work together in cause and effect sequences of physical and chemical processes to ensure our health and well-being. When we start to control our nutritional intake to lose weight, we interfere with the delicate sequences of our physiological processes, and impose on our bodies unnecessary stress. Thus we limit our natural mechanisms which are designed to promote and enhance our experience of life. By limiting our food, we limit our ability to reach our optimum potential.

Insights Into Losing Weight

Most people want to lose weight fast. Once people hear about a fast way to lose weight, they try it with no regard to its health consequences. Even the most learned people who know everything there is to know about weight loss often fall into this trap of attempting to lose weight by reducing calories and starving themselves. There are more than a thousand different theories and diet plans that show you how to starve yourself and lose weight fast. Like innocent lambs going to the slaughter, many people listen to these money making schemes and risk their health and well-being for the sake of their vanity. They want to believe the false promises and guarantees that they can lose ten pounds in three weeks or sixteen pounds in two weeks. Diet gimmicks like these are the reason many people <u>gain</u> weight not lose it!

The mechanics of burning body fat are far more complicated than these fast weight loss programs tell us. It is not as simple a formula as:

Exercise + Restricted Calorie Diet = Permanent Weight-loss

I will show you that this formula changes our metabolism and makes us susceptible to weight gain. Our bodies react to lowered food intake by lowering demand on energy needs, and burning less fuel to do work. This is one sure way to increase body fat. All quick weight loss diet plans, *interrupt and retard body metabolism.*

Almost all diets that promise quick weight loss are

low calorie diets and they do not work. We might lose a few pounds in the initial ten days or so of the diet, but when we start eating normally, we gain back all the weight we have lost and a little more. Although we have large amounts of energy stored as fat in our body, we cannot live off our fat for too long. We must provide ourselves with nutrients on a regular basis. One of the reasons that we must eat regularly is that our brain cannot utilize fat, brain cells can only utilize a sugar based energy released in the blood as glucose. In chapter 7 we will discuss how our bodies utilize their energy, and under what conditions our bodies will be able to burn fat. We will also find out how important it is to ensure a steady energy supply to the brain so our brain cells will not starve and slow down our metabolism making us feel tired, depressed, and grouchy. On the other hand, in chapter 19 we will see how eating too much sugar can cause problems. We will see how our bodies are sensitive to sugar, and how eating sugar, or even tasting anything sweet, stops our bodies from burning fat. It is important to know how body mechanisms work, so we may be able to work with our bodies and not against them.

Our body mechanisms work together for the benefit of the whole body. The body as a whole ensures the survival of each of our organs, tissues, and cells. We can say the body is a unit working together, "one for all and all for one". In attempting to lose weight by controlling our calorie intake we are focusing on, and manipulating, only one aspect and one process of our body mechanisms. This throws all the other body mechanisms out of kilter. The less we interfere with our bodily processes, the more our bodies will be able to function and excel as they were designed to. Just like a machine needs all of its parts assembled and working together simultaneously to function properly, so the human body is specifically organized to carry out our life-sustaining processes.

In chapter 4 we will learn about the various neurochemicals and endorphins that are involved in regulating all body mechanisms. Neurochemicals and endorphins are released in our bodies and make us experience pleasure and feel good. The good feelings that we experience compel us to pursue the activities that promote well-being in all aspects of our lives and we innately learn what we must do to become healthy and fit. In Chapter 12 we will see how our bodies innately learn which nutrients we require, when, and how much. Also we will explore how our sensations and feelings help us recognize and chose the types of foods which contain the nutrients that we require. By responding to our innate requests, we develop the ability to cue into the foods that contain the nutrients that are needed by each and every cell. By not responding to our innate requests which are conveyed to us in sensations of hunger, cravings, and satiation, we will fail to develop our innate mechanisms that control eating and we will not be able to meet our body needs. As a result we may overeat and become fat or undereat and still become fat because of lowered metabolism.

Why Do Some People Become Fat?

The traditional answer to this question is that people gain weight when they consume more energy than they burn. Although this is true, it does not mean that fat people eat more than thin people. Perhaps fat people use less energy than they consume.

Energy intake must equal energy output to obtain a neutral energy balance. When the calories obtained from the food that we eat are equal to what we expend in metabolic energy, there will not be any weight gain. Traditionally, it is assumed that there are three ways in which the body can react with regard to food intake.

1. If the energy in food we eat equals the amount of energy we expend, then body weight will remain constant.

2. If the amount of energy in food we eat is more than the amount of the energy we expend, the extra energy intake is stored as body fat.

3. If the energy derived from food eaten is less than the body's immediate need, the body will use its stored energy to supply energy needs, causing weight loss.

We must remember that our body mechanisms do more than just burn the calories we consume. Our bodies are complex physiological entities with their own systems and organization. Our metabolic functions possess a tenacity and "wisdom" designed to preserve and sustain our lives and well-being *automatically*. The consumption and the use of energy by our bodies are not a simple balancing out of energy intake to energy output, but rather are complex processes aimed at sustaining life and the well-being of the body as a whole. Therefore our attempts to consciously regulate our energy intake to our energy output to maintain a desired weight often do not work and disrupt our innate body processes.

Energy Needs in The Body

Body cells require energy to carry out specialized functions that are essential for the survival of the body as a whole. The energy used by our body cells is provided by the food that we eat. Nutrients are substances that provide essential nourishment for maintenance of life. These include vitamins, minerals, and the molecules of fats, carbohydrates, and proteins that contain carbon atoms which are held together by chemical energy bonds. These molecules are separated from each other during biochemical activities in the cells and the energy from the bonds is released. The energy that is released from the splitting of molecules is then harvested and used by our body cells immediately, or we store this energy as fat or glycogen which we use later when needed.

Energy cannot be created or destroyed, so says the law of conservation of energy. The energy that is released from food constitutes the same energy that can be expended. Energy expended in the body falls under two categories. Energy expended by the muscles to mobilize the body in the external environment is under voluntary control. Energy expended for internal body functions to do all internal activities is under involuntary control.

Internal work includes two types of activities:

1. Work that includes skeletal muscles which are not related to movement of the muscles in the outside environment. This work for example, includes the maintenance of posture and shivering.

2. Work involved in maintaining all internal activities which must go on all the time to sustain life, such as pumping blood through the blood vessels, breathing, growth and repair of tissue, and all other metabolic reactions in the body.

Not all the energy harnessed from food molecules is used to perform biological work. The energy that is not used to energize biological work is used as heat energy. Only half the energy we receive from food is transferred to biological work energy. The other 50% is lost as heat energy immediately. Then half of the energy used in biological work is also released as heat during the process of doing work. It means that 75% of the energy taken from food is used up in heat energy and only 25% is used to perform work in various biological processes. The biological work performed is eventually converted to heat. The rate at which the body uses energy to perform its biological work is measured in units of heat.

The basic unit of heat is a calorie, which is the amount of heat energy required to raise the temperature of one cubic centimeter, (or one gram) of water one degree Celsius. This unit is too small to discuss the magnitude of heat required in the human body. Nutritionists speak of kilocalories, where one kilocalorie is equivalent to 1000 calories. Four calories of heat are released from one gram of carbohydrate when it is burned by the body or even in a laboratory by a heat source.

The amount of energy that is required by our bodies when we are at rest is referred to as the basal metabolic rate (BMR). This is measured by the amount of oxygen we use when we are at rest.

Balancing Energy Intake To Energy Output

Weight is maintained when energy received from food is equal to energy expenditure by our bodies. Many weight-conscious people have learned how to balance their dietary needs to their energy output, and can monitor all the food that enters their mouths. They have learned to plan and prepare their meals using their knowledge of caloric and nutritional requirements. They measure their weight by a scale and their body fat by pinching various parts of their body on a regular basis. They may even use very sophisticated body fat measuring devices that work using ultrasound. Besides regulating their diet and measuring body fat, many weight-conscious people participate in exercise programs to keep fit. Some people do a marvelous job and can maintain a constant desired body weight, relying solely on self-discipline and ample time to exercise. Some have been successful in maintaining their weight this way. Diet and exercise have become the accepted foundation for weight loss and healthy living.

There is no question that healthy bodies come about from a healthy lifestyle. However once people lose the desired amount of weight, they continue to remain in a "constant battle of the bulge". Invariably, many people who attempt to reduce their weight by dieting and exercise, will eventually gain back all the weight they have lost and in some cases, end up with more weight than when they started. There are a few heroes who conquer this battle of weight gain vs. weight loss and remain victorious. However, many of us struggle every day with every morsel of food. We constantly question ourselves, "Should I eat it? Should I not? Oh...what the heck!" The minute we let our guard down and indulge a little, we gain back any weight that we may have struggled so hard to shed. Why do we have to stay in a constant battle with our weight? Are there no other choices?

For answers we must look at some clinical research. Scientists experimented on two groups of rats which were not subjected to overeating or undereating practices. They chose rats who were normal eaters, and fed them supermarket junk such as cookies and potato chips, and increased their caloric intake by about 80%. Despite an 80% increase in calorie intake, weight gain was only 27% higher than that of diet controlled animals. Their resting oxygen consumption was consistently higher than that of controlled animals. The increase in oxygen consumption was not due to increased physical activity because the animals were housed in pairs in small cages, meaning that their metabolic rate was higher than diet controled animals (Rothwell and

Stock, 1979).

Studies on human subjects showed similar findings indicating that metabolic rate rises when food is not restricted. Volunteers overate by 1600 calories per day, for a period of ten days. At the end of the ten days their metabolic rate had increased by 22% (Welle, Nair, and Campbell 1989)

It has been found that a single meal or a stimuli associated with eating can cause a rise in the metabolic rate. LeBlanc and Cabanac (1989) placed human subjects in a chamber so that their oxygen consumption could be monitored, and their metabolic rate could be determined. They reported that eating a sugar pie, tasting it and chewing it, then spitting it out, caused an increase in their metabolic rate. They also found that the metabolic rate increased even when subjects went through the motions of eating, moving their hands to their mouth, making chewing and swallowing motions. The metabolic rate increases because the body is preparing to receive food. Digestive juices are released in preparation to digest the food about to be eaten, hormones and insulin are released to metabolize the nutrients absorbed. All this extra activity causes an increase in the basal metabolic rate.

Many people, after battling with their weight for many years, reluctantly succumb to the idea that they might have to remain overweight for the rest of their lives. They can no longer torture themselves with dieting and deprive themselves of eating what they want. They stop dieting and eat at liberty, whatever and whenever they feel like it, enjoying their lives. To their surprise, they begin to maintain a fairly steady weight. The phenomenon occurs because their metabolic rate rises and they start to burn more calories when they start eating the foods they want.

Evidence is beginning to show that people who are successfully controlling their weight, in some instances, take in more calories than unsuccessful overweight individuals. These people seem to have bodies that are able to adjust to a constant weight with little conscious effort. They instinctively know what to eat, when to eat, and how much.

Do We Innately Know What To Eat, When, and How Much?

The average adult does maintain a constant weight over a long period of time. When we overeat, our bodies raise our metabolisms and we start to burn more calories. This indicates that there is a mechanism in the body that checks the balance between energy intake and energy output. Some studies have found that the body adjusts its metabolism to meet energy supply conditions. For instance, when food intake is reduced for a few weeks to lose weight, and after losing ten pounds or so, the body lowers its metabolism and the person reaches a plateau and stops losing weight for a while. The same phenomenon occurs when people start to eat more to gain weight. Their body metabolism rises and they burn more calories and their weight gain reaches a plateau.

In 1928, Clara Davis, a pediatrician, conducted an experiment in Chicago. She placed fifteen infants on a self serve diet, which allowed them to choose their own meals. Infants in this experiment were newly weaned from their mothers' milk. They were placed in a hospital setting, away from their mothers. A wide variety of food items listed in table one, were served to the babies.

A nurse was available to observe and give to the children whatever they requested or pointed to. Nurses did not interfere with making any choices for the children. They merely observed and helped children to reach and hold the food as required. Pureed food items were presented to the children on a tray. Each type of food was presented to the babies in a separate dish. Even salt was placed in a separate dish and not added to the food. If the child finished a particular food item, the portion of that food item was increased in the next serving. This experiment was undertaken to study what children would choose to eat for themselves. The study was done over a six-month period.

A Sample Menu For Self Served Diet Experiment

Meats: beef, lamb chicken, offal liver, kidneys, brains, bone marrow.

Fish: haddock.

Fruits: apples, oranges, bananas, tomatoes, peaches, pineapple.

Vegetables: lettuce, cabbage, spinach, cauliflower, peas, beets, carrots, turnip, potatoes.

Cereals: ground whole wheat, oatmeal, barley, cornmeal, rye.

Other: Jelly, Milk, Eggs.

Sea salt.

All foods were finely chopped or pureed to prevent choking.

Table 1

The results were surprising. Dr. Davis reported that the children thrived on their self served meals. They enjoyed their food and had healthy appetites. The food they chose to eat over the six month period was nutritionally well balanced and the children were healthy. However, these children achieved this balanced diet by unconventional means which Dr. Davis described as "a dietitian's nightmare". During the first few weeks the children tasted their food at random, swallowing some and spitting out others, expressing surprise to some tastes and dislike to others. As the weeks went by, the children started to recognize particular foods, and began to make clear choices. They reached for specific foods and ignored others. They ate about three solid food items for each meal. Their meals did not conform to traditional child's meals. Breakfast, for instance, consisted of orange juice and pureed liver, while supper consisted of eggs, banana, and milk. They showed temporary preferences which lasted for several weeks at a time, as if they had a series of cravings for specific foods. Although their diets were balanced on a long-term basis, they were not balanced on a daily basis, let alone in a single meal. Dr. Davis speculated that their cravings were caused by the changing nutritional needs of a growing child. Several observations were made, suggesting that the children were showing dietary awareness. They all ate salt regularly, despite their coughing, making faces, sputtering and crying while eating the salt. One child was suffering from rickets before joining the study. A container of cod liver oil was made available to him on his tray. This child drank the cod liver oil and all the milk that was placed on his tray during the first three months of the study. After three months he stopped drinking the cod liver oil. Testing revealed that his rickets had healed. He appeared to have had the appetite for cod liver oil while his body needed it. The child did not care for it after he was cured. Dr. Davis observed that the children in her study instinctively chose what their bodies required.

Another study was undertaken by Dr. Samuel Fomon during the late 1970's on infants who were bottle fed. The purpose of this study was to find out if babies would drink more if their milk had less energy in it. (Similar experiments with rats had shown that rats eat greater quantities of food when their diet contains less calories.) Dr. Fomon diluted the formulas given to the mothers to feed to their babies. He provided the mothers with three different strengths of baby formula. One had 35 calories per 100 cc, the second had 66 calories per 100 cc, and a third mix had 133 calories per 100 cc. He weighed the formulas before and after feeding and calculated the caloric intake for each feeding. Dr. Fomon discovered some surprising results. Babies over six months old were able to regulate calorie intake. Babies given diluted formula drank more than babies given concentrated formula in their feeding. He also reported that babies before the age of six months showed very few signs indicating that they can regulate their caloric intake. When babies reached six months, they appeared to have more mature dietary regulation mechanisms.

Sir Walter Canon, the renowned physiologist, in his book "The Wisdom Of The Body" (1939), discusses how our bodies have mechanisms in place that cope automatically with dangerous and life-threatening situations. For example, during intense emotions the body reacts and increases blood glucose and fatty acids to carry out actions requiring more vigor and strength such as running faster and lifting heavier loads. Other changes that may occur during stressful situations include lowering of blood pressure, or increasing levels of insulin to speed up metabolic activities. Canon promoted the idea that the body, if left alone, will do what is best to cope with existing situations.

There is no question that our bodies have an internal signaling device for stocking up depleted nutritional substances by initiating hunger and cravings. These signaling mechanisms are designed to assist the person to select the appropriate food needed by the body cells. Just as there are mechanisms to initiate eating, there are also mechanisms that initiate satiety and cause cessation of eating after the required quantities of nutrients are consumed.

The Phenomenon Of Craving and The Mechanisms Which Control Eating

We have mechanisms in our bodies that trigger sensations of hunger to remind us that we should eat. And, we tend to forget that we also have mechanisms in our bodies that trigger feelings of satiation. When we eat in response to our feelings of hunger and satiation, we feel refreshed and satisfied. On the other hand if we do not eat when we feel hungry, we start to feel tired and weak. Hunger sensations are internal feelings that make us think of eating. When we stop eating in response to our feelings of satiety, we feel content. However if we continue to eat beyond the point of satiation, the discomfort of a distended stomach may be the only thing that can stop us from eating any more. By being aware of and responding to our feelings of hunger and satiation we learn when to eat and when to stop eating automatically and effortlessly. If only we would make the effort to respond to these feelings instead of trying to control and interfere with them.

When our nutritive stores are depleted, we develop a desire to eat, and our hunger persists until our nutritive stores are replenished. When we eat the same type of food for a while, we lose our appetite for that food because our nutritional reserves are replenished with that particular nutrient. This explains why sometimes we like to eat a certain thing and other times we do not have a taste for it. The precise mechanisms with which our depletion of nutritive stores affects hunger is not well understood, although it is known that decreased levels of glucose in body fluid are associated with one's hunger. Usually, when blood glucose is depleted other nutrients are also depleted (Sherwood, 1990).

A perfect example of how our bodies can regulate our food intake is the phenomenon of craving. A craving is not merely a feeling of hunger but rather a compelling desire for a specific food item. No matter how much that person eats other foods, the craving for that specific food remains until the craved food is eaten. For example, one pregnant woman described her craving experience for chalk like this:

> "I wanted to eat chalk. I wanted to eat white powdery chalk. I felt an urge to lick something that tasted like chalk. My husband would not go and get me some chalk. So I went out to find some chalk from a nearby school. It was late at night...the schools were closed, so I went to an open convenience store instead, hoping that they might have some chalk. As I entered the store, I saw an advertisement with a picture of a cold glass of milk. I realized what I was craving for was milk. Suddenly, I felt the urge to drink a glass of cold skim milk, and forgot all about chalk. I was not much of a milk drinker before, but on that day at 3:00 a.m. there was nothing more satisfying or better tasting than that cold glass of milk. After drinking milk I felt very happy."

Most people describe their craving experience as a sudden thought that pops to their mind and a sense of urgency to eat specific foods. Some people can visualize the food they desire. Others can smell and taste the food they are craving. Usually people crave for foods that they have not eaten for a while. In the pregnant woman's case, her body probably needed calcium since she was four months pregnant at the time. Chalk is very rich in calcium. She might have eaten chalk as a child and recalled the taste when there was a shortage of calcium in her body. Maybe she subconsciously knew that she needed calcium. Maybe she knowingly replaced her craving for chalk with milk. The most important point here is that her body initiated the need to eat something containing calcium, and she was compelled to satisfy that need by her conscious action. When her body was short of calcium, the craving for chalk was triggered. Upon seeing the picture of a glass of milk, she also remembered the taste of milk which could satisfy her physical need.

Scientists have suspected for a long time that the hypothalamus, which is the part of the brain that controls the autonomic functions of the body (functions that are outside our control), contains the control centers of hunger and satiety. We all know that a person has no control over his feelings of hunger or satiety. Although we tend to exercise control by eating or not eating, we cannot make our hunger go away without eating. Something in our body makes us conscious that we are hungry and should start to eat, and when we've had enough to eat, something in our body informs us that we feel full and should stop eating.

Scientists believed that the hypothalamus housed two centers for controlling hunger and satiety. In the 1950's, scientists studying rats located a pair of nerve clusters in the lateral regions of the hypothalamus that initiate hunger and named it the feeding or appetite center. They also located another pair of nerve clusters in the more medial region of the hypothalamus and named this the satiety center. Many experiments have been carried out on these two centers and the findings demonstrate that stimulation of the feeding centers causes the animal to start eating and destruction of the feeding centers causes the animal to starve to death. On the other hand, the stimulation of the satiety centers causes the animal to refuse to eat, and the destruction of the cells in the satiety centers causes the animal to keep eating causing severe obesity.

Himmi, Boyer, and Orsini (1988) discovered that many neurons in the hypothalamus change their firing rate in response to the fluctuation of blood glucose levels in the blood supplied to the brain. Burton, Rolls, and Mora (1976) found that some neurons in the hypothalamus respond to the sight or the taste of specific food only if the animal is hungry. Rolls, Murzi, Yaxley, Thorpe, and Simpson (1986) discovered that the firing rate of these neurons was related to specific satiety. When animals had enough of a specific food to eat, they lost their appetite for that specific food and neurons in their brain stopped reacting when they saw or smelled that food. These studies indicate that our bodies have mechanisms for controlling eating, and the brain reacts to specific foods only if we are hungry. After we eat enough of any type of food, we will start to dislike that food for a while, and neurons in our hypothalamus stop becoming excited by the sight or the smell of that food. Conversely when we are hungry, certain neurons in the hypothalamus begin to fire at the sight or smell of the foods that our nutritive reserves require. (It is also quite logical to assume that our neurons become excited when we think of the food that our bodies require without actually seeing or smelling it, even though this is not demonstrated in an experiment.)

Although we have specific areas in our brain that control our hunger and satiation, mechanisms which trigger eating are governed by many other factors and inputs from various parts of our bodies which synchronize our body's activities to the various time of the day. Various neurochemicals, proteins, and hormones are released in the body periodically throughout the day which control body organs and glands telling them to start or to stop their actions; such as the production of insulin and gastric juices which trigger hunger sensations. Thus our hunger and satiation are also synchronized by the time of the day and not just by the nutrients needed in the body. We will discuss this further in Chapter 14 on Biological Rhythms.

Chapter 2

Food and The Body

The Dietary Needs of The Body

What would happen if we did not drink milk when we wanted to drink milk and we drank a glass of juice, or a glass of water instead? Let us say we are on a diet and we have already had our share of milk for that day so we drink some juice instead. The craving for milk is most likely triggered by a need for calcium in our bodies. By drinking something else, would the requisition for calcium go away? No, not until the stores for calcium in our bodies become replenished. The orange juice has some calcium, but not in the same quantities as a glass of milk, and water has small traces of minerals but no other nutrients. The orange juice might not satisfy our need for calcium and we will start to nibble here and there, searching for something, waiting for the next meal. What we really want is a glass of milk. Why can't we have a glass of milk? If by chance we happen to nibble on some cheese, then we will be in luck. Cheese contains as much calcium as milk and satisfies our need for calcium. Meanwhile, all the other nutrients eaten during our search for calcium are extra foods that we did not need to have. All extra foods that we eat, if not immediately used are stored in our bodies as fat.

Our bodies need energy to carry out work and main-tain our temperature. We need proteins to repair and build cells and for growth. Minerals are necessary to maintain fluid balance and cellular activities. We need water to dissolve all nutrients including minerals and oxygen and transport them to all our body cells. Water flushes all residues which have been produced by meta-bolic activities, and replaces moisture evaporated from our skin surface and expelled by our lungs. Vitamins act as catalysts in cell metabolism and are required in the building of cell structures. Our bodies are wise and resourceful; we can juggle our resources in accordance with our priorities. For example, if there is a shortage of water in our bodies our circulatory system draws some water from our gastrointestinal tract. When there is a shortage of glucose energy, our bodies strip proteins from our muscle cells to burn for fuel. We use all three types of food nutrients, proteins, carbohydrates, and fats interchangeably to satisfy our energy needs. When the supply of energy is diminished, our bodies burn whatever is available. Our bodies have a good sense of economy. We never waste any nutrients. Our bodies convert all unused energy into fat and store it for fu-ture use. Nutrients are used in our bodies on an ongo-ing basis, and they must be replaced. Our bodies are equipped with mechanisms that trigger hunger sensa-tions and cravings to make us eat the nutrients that we require at the cellular level. Why do we have to con-trol our hunger and wait until it is time to eat? Why can't we eat what we feel we want to eat? When we do not respond to our innate eating requests and train ourselves to do otherwise, we often short-change ourselves. Even if we use a state of the art computer with sensitive, elaborate software and the most sophisticated input data (there is such a computer program available on the market), such a computer will not be able to calculate our nutritional needs because our needs vary according to physical and emotional changes we experience from day to day. How will this computer know how we feel? People do not come in standard specifications. Even if we have a constant height and weight, our energy requirements change from day to day.

Meeting our dietary needs does not have to be a complicated science. Our bodies already have more advanced computing mechanisms, the likes of which are yet to be duplicated by technology. Our bodies know what we need and how to satisfy those needs. We need to learn how to respond to our feelings and cues; the various sensations and cravings that our bodies are constantly relating to us. What we need is to re-learn how to focus and relate to ourselves, and how to read our own feelings. Of course, there was a time when we were little babies and we knew how to relate to our feelings and sensations, but as we grew older we learned to ignore those feelings, not only in our eating matters but in many other areas beyond the scope of this book.

There is always a constant calling in our bodies for one type of nutrient or another. Our craving mechanisms are triggered when we start to use our reserves. We can manage quite well with the nutrients that we have on hand so we need not worry if some nutrients arrive late as long as nutrients arrive before the depletion of the reserves.

Our bodies keep limited quantities of nutrients on hand for immediate use and trigger hunger sensations before our reserves are depleted. Most of the energy from food consumed in a given day is stored in the liver and perhaps used the next day. When the reserves in the liver are full, the body changes the structures of carbohydrates and proteins and stores them as fat which is used maybe in two or three weeks.

We need to drink water every day. Water is always balanced out in our bodies by the action of the kidneys. When we drink more water than required, our kidneys excrete the excess water in the urine. When we do not drink enough water, our kidneys reduce the amount of water removed from the body, and our urine becomes concentrated. Shortages of water result in damage to our kidneys, blocking our filtration system. Most other nutrients are also needed continuously, however, we maintain enough reserves in our cells and liver that are used first, and we feel hungry when we start to use our reserves.

We do not have to be overly concerned if we do not eat all the nutrients that are recommended for us to eat in a day. These daily requirements are guides. If we do not eat all that is recommended for us to eat in one day, we can perhaps eat them the next day. The important thing is that we eat what our bodies need to carry out their functions, and so we must replenish our reserves before they become depleted.

When we practice eating the foods that our innate eating mechanisms requisition, we accustom ourselves to become responsive to our needs. When we learn to automatically and effortlessly eat the foods that our body cells require, our nutritional reserves will remain full. We will then be able to eat discriminately, choosing only the foods that we need. When several signals trigger hunger sensation, calling for a multitude of nutrients required by our bodies, we will not be able to discriminate what we want to eat. We will then feel a need to eat everything that is available to us.

For example, regardless of how much protein, fat and sugar there is in the body, if there are shortages of calcium, iron, other minerals, or vitamins, the body will trigger a sensation of hunger and a craving for a specific food which is rich in the minerals and vitamins that we require.

Most people who refrain from eating in response to their innate requests of craving and hunger, and eat according to various guidelines and planned menus, often find themselves unsatisfied when they eat their specified and rationed meals. They feel unsatisfied because although they have met the specific nutritional requirements of their menu, they have not met the specific nutritional requirements of their *bodies*. They keep resisting their hunger and ignoring their cravings, until they eventually give up and start to binge, eating indiscriminately.

When we eat foods our bodies have not called for we still digest and absorb them, and if we do not need them we store them as fat. When we eat in response to feeling hungry, we will be able to know the foods that we are craving, and learn to discriminate and choose the foods required by our bodies at that specific time.

But when people eat according to diet menus they will eat all sorts of things on a "hit or miss" basis, hoping to meet the needs of their bodies, and if their reserves are full momentarily, they will, much to their dismay, store their diet menu as fat.

All foods although rich in one sort of nutrient or another, contain a variety of all other groups of nutrients, minerals, vitamins, carbohydrates, proteins, and fats. The innocent lettuce contains molecules of fat, proteins, and carbohydrates. For example, one slice of bread contains two grams of protein, three or four grams of carbohydrates and some fat. One egg contains four grams of protein, and twelve grams of carbohydrates and fat. A glass of milk is rich in calcium, and contains protein, carbohydrates, and fat. When we crave for the specific taste of a certain food, our desire stems from needing one or more of the nutrients found in that food. By eating the food that we have craved our need is satisfied. Of course there will be other nutrients in the food that we have craved for that our bodies have no momentary use for. These extra nutrients will be stored as fat for future use. Sometimes cravings are satisfied by eating other foods that also contain the nutrients requested. For example the craving for spinach, which is rich in iron, can be easily replaced by eating a steak which is also rich in iron, the other nutrients in the steak being stored for later use.

Our preferences depend on what experiences we have had with food. They also depend on what we see and smell and how we have been introduced to certain foods. Thus, it is important to eat and teach ourselves taste, texture, and how our hunger is satisfied by the various foods that are economical and are easily attainable in the part of the world we live. It is wise to learn about the nutritional content of our food so we develop a taste for foods that contain less fat, because our bodies convert all nutrients whether carbohydrates or proteins, into fat when there is no immediate use for these nutrients in our bodies.

Therefore, it is essential to become nutritionally wise and train ourselves to make wise choices in the foods we eat. It is essential that we learn to develop a taste for a variety of foods that are cheap, nutritious, and available to us. We must learn how to prepare our foods so that all their nutrients are preserved and our money does not go down the drain along with the vitamins and minerals. Most of all, it is wise to learn about ourselves and how to be responsive to our sensations of hunger, craving, and satiation. We must earnestly respond to these innate feelings and develop innate eating skills according to our nutritional needs. By eating to satisfy our hunger and cravings, we will improve and develop the ability to choose the foods our bodies need. When we meet our needs, we will not overeat. We need to learn to reflect on our emotions and moods and to learn about ourselves, so we can differentiate between the need to eat to satisfy a physical hunger, and those eating habits which we use to attain emotional gratification.

Nutrition is the study of nutrients in foods and how the body handles these nutrients. Proper nutrition is maintained when we take into consideration the body's nutritional requirements at the cellular level, how our body reacts with the various foods that we eat, and the enjoyment we receive from eating.

The Major Groups of Nutrients

All energy required in our bodies is derived from carbohydrates, fats, and proteins. Figure 1 shows the basic forms of carbohydrates, fats, and proteins.

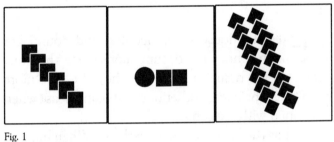

Fig. 1

Carbohydrate   Protein   Fat

Carbohydrates

Carbohydrates are composed of simple sugars. These sugars are made up of carbon, hydrogen, and oxygen atoms. These atoms are constructed in different configurations to form three types of carbohydrates. For our purposes, all carbohydrates are converted into blood sugar which has six carbon molecules. Every time oxygen unites with a chain of this six carbon molecule, it splits it into two molecules with three carbons in each, releasing energy in the process. If a three-car-

41

bon molecule is not needed, it can join back together with another three-carbon molecule and stay in the blood as glucose. When three-carbon carbohydrate molecules further break and lose one more carbon atom they turn into fat structures and cannot be used as glucose again, and brain cells will not be able to utilize their energy. When carbohydrates and proteins are not required in the body, they are converted to fat molecules and stored in the body in fat cells.

Fat

Fat cells house fat molecules, and pound per pound, not only occupy more space than any other type of tissue in the body, they also give more than twice the energy other nutrients can release when combined with oxygen.

Fat has the largest chain of carbons. When burned, it releases more energy than carbohydrates or proteins. Although fat is constructed of carbon, hydrogen, and oxygen molecules, the configuration of a fat molecule differs from that of a carbohydrate or protein molecule. Fat contains eighteen atoms of carbon in one molecule of fatty acid.

Fat tissue is found almost everywhere in the body, under the skin, over the muscles, between muscles, around the heart and the kidneys, all around the bowels, and over the blood vessels. Fat is stored in almost all the places that are not filled by other body tissues. Sometimes it is also found inside the blood vessels. When fat molecules are deposited inside the blood vessel walls they restrict blood flow to the tissues and muscles the vessel is supplying. Restricted blood supply to muscles causes cramping, and obstruction of blood supply causes the death of muscle tissue because nutrients cannot reach the cells and waste by-products cannot be removed. When fat cells cause restriction of blood supply to the heart muscle, it results in cramping of the heart muscle and the person will experience chest pains that disappear when resting. This is known as *angina*. But when fat deposits cause blockage of blood supply to the heart muscle causing suffocation of the muscle cells, then the blocks of cells not receiving adequate nutrients and oxygen will die, this is referred to as a *heart attack*.

It is not healthy to become fat because it causes many complications besides the extra strain of the sheer weight of the excess fat that muscles have to carry around. For every pound of body fat, there is the equivalent of one mile of blood vessels that the heart has to pump blood through. Imagine how much harder our heart has to work if we accumulate ten pounds of extra fat!

Many people who have large bones and big muscles will normally weigh much more than people who have small builds. People who have more muscle content are heavier, but are not necessarily fat. Also, people who develop their muscles, improve their blood circulation, taking the strain off the heart. The scales cannot tell the truth about who is fat and who is not. The scales can only tell who is heavier. Muscular people with large bones will weigh more on the scale regardless of their height! It is important that people take their body frame and musculature into consideration before they assume that they are fat or unhealthy.

Weight charts and other statistical data have been proven to be wrong. These generalized statistical charts stipulating weight according to height, body frame size, and gender are the reason many people are fat today. Many people who had ideal weights in relation to their height, and body make-up have desperately dieted to achieve the weights these statistical charts claimed to be ideal weights for healthy people. Their efforts to lose weight and meet the stipulations of these charts have rendered them susceptible to gain weight.

Men need to worry more about their weight than women in terms of health consequences, because there is a difference in where each gender carries their fat deposits. Men carry most of their fat reserves around their abdomen and chest, encumbering the breathing muscles and the heart. Women carry their fat reserves on their thighs and buttocks encumbering their agility and speed. Men need to be more concerned about becoming fat since their accumulation of fat interferes more with their vital organs.

Any fat molecule consumed in the diet is directly deposited into the various fat reserves in the body, enlarging the fat cells. When new fat molecules enter a fat cell they push out the existing fat molecules already in the cells into the blood stream. Therefore, the fat in the fat cells is in constant flux, and 50% of it is exchanged about every eight days. After eating fat in our diet, our body quickly removes the extra surge of fat found in the blood stream and regulates its release into the blood stream after carbohydrates and sugar are metabolized. Sugars that are eaten in a meal must be utilized first before the body will use fat for energy. Later, in Chapter 7, we will see how this becomes important in bringing about the ideal conditions to allow our bodies to burn fat. The reason our bodies utilize carbohydrates and sugars first, is because once a sugar molecule is converted to a fat molecule it cannot be converted back to sugar again. So in any meal containing fat and sugar, the fat is deposited in the fat cells directly while sugar is utilized first. Our body mechanisms are smart and efficiently utilize energy. Why bother converting sugar to fat? It is less work for our bodies to use sugar as sugar and store the fat which does not need any converting. Also once sugar is converted to fat it will have to burn as fat and cannot be converted to sugar again, so our brain cells which need sugar and cannot utilize fat will not benefit much.

Fat is digested and absorbed more slowly than carbohydrates and proteins. The absorption of fat takes place in the small intestine. The pancreatic enzyme, lipase, breaks fat down into absorbable units called fatty acids. Bile released from the gall bladder converts fat into an emulsion that consists of many small fat droplets which are able to mix with the water based nature of the rest of the food in the stomach known as *chyme*. Bile salts exert a detergent action similar to that of the dish soap you use to cut grease. This speeds up the digestion and absorption of fat in the small intestine. Fat is then absorbed into the lymphatic vessels and not directly into the blood. The lymphatic vessel then empties into the portal vein that goes directly to the liver and fatty acids are transported from the liver to fat cells.

Although fat is the most despised part of our bodies and is blamed for everything that goes wrong, body fat is useful and important to us. It is our only constant, dependable energy source and uninterrupted energy is so vital to life. Fat is our only means of storing large quantities of uninterrupted energy. At the slightest shortage of energy many important functions are sacrificed to maintain our energy supply. To go totally without energy means death. *It is no surprise then, that our bodies become prone to stockpiling fat when subjected to reduced energy intake during dieting.*

Fat is necessary to our body, and in an average person, fat constitutes 60% of the body's ongoing energy supply when at rest, and far more during exercise, especially if one has well-developed muscles. Fatty tissues around the various organs form a pad that protects the organs from physical shock. Cell membranes are mainly composed of fat molecules. Hormones, bile, and vitamin D are all structured from fat molecules. This does not mean we need to choose to eat fat in our diet. The body makes its own fat from unused carbohydrates and protein molecules.

The body stores its reserve energy in the form of fat because it is the most economical and efficient way to do so. It is light, compact, and releases the most energy when burned. One gram of fat yields nine calories of energy while one gram of carbohydrates yields four calories and one gram of protein yields seven calories.

It is important that we understand the way the body utilizes energy reserves, (discussed extensively in Chapter 7) and the important role fat has in securing a dependable energy source for the metabolic activities of our bodies. Understanding how we use fat for our energy helps us to work with our bodies and allow ourselves to utilize our body fat.

Many people strive so hard to "get rid of their fat", but we just cannot get rid of it. We can only help ourselves to bring about the conditions in our bodies that are conducive to *burning* fat instead of *stockpiling* it. We have to understand how our bodies use energy, and what factors are involved in our physiological processes that allow us to utilize our fat. When all our physiological conditions are geared toward burning fat, then our bodies will gladly burn fat for our energy needs.

Proteins

Proteins are molecules composed of atoms of carbon, hydrogen, and nitrogen. They differ from fats and carbohydrates because of their nitrogen atoms. The protein that we eat in food cannot be directly used by our bodies. All proteins taken in from the various foods are broken down into molecular structures called amino acids. The proteins in the diet supply the amino acids from which our bodies make our own proteins. To construct different kinds of body proteins we need nine essential amino acids. They are called "essential" because all the nine different types of amino acids must be present simultaneously so we can make new body proteins. Even if a meal contains eight of the nine essential amino acids, the body cannot use those eight. Our body enzymes will strip the nitrogen from the eight amino acids absorbed from the meal and expel them from the body as urea. The remaining carbon and hydrogen molecules from such a meal are then converted to glucose and will become fat if there is not an immediate need for glucose. It is important that proteins in a meal contain at least nine essential amino acids, to allow the body to construct its own proteins. A meal that contains nine essential amino acids is referred to as containing complete protein.

Egg protein has been designated as the reference protein for the purpose of measuring protein quality, and is assigned a biological value of 100 by the food and agriculture organization of the United Nations. This means that 100% of the amino acids from an egg can be converted to body proteins. Other animal or vegetable proteins have a lesser value than 100, meaning that not all the amino acids from these sources can be converted to body proteins.

Most animal source proteins contain all the essential amino acids required to make body proteins. Non-animal proteins that are found in vegetables, seeds, legumes, and nuts are incomplete proteins. By eating a combination of incomplete proteins in one meal one can obtain all the essential amino acids and the meal then can be considered to contain complete proteins. The rule of thumb for vegetarians to ensure the consumption of all the nine essential amino acids, is to include a combination of incomplete proteins from one white and one yellow grain or vegetable source in one meal. For example, combinations of corn and potatoes, or lentils and rice, or chick peas and rice eaten together will ensure the presence of all the amino acids needed to make body proteins. When any of these foods are eaten separately, the chances are that not all the amino acids required will be present in one meal. Our bodies will then use the grains for energy or store them as fat, instead of being able to derive the amino acids from them that are necessary for our bodies' own protein-making machinery.

What Happens To The Food After We Eat It?

The foods we eat are first ground and pulverized in the mouth by chewing. Then various enzymes and digestive juices are poured and mixed with the food during digestion. Digestion starts in the mouth with salivary amylase which breaks down and digests sugar molecules. Then juices from the stomach and pancreas, and bile from the gall bladder are emptied into the digestive system to continue digesting the food as it passes through our intestinal tract.

The food is churned in the stomach with hydrochloric acid and is broken down into smaller absorbable molecules, that are diffused throughout the blood vessel walls into the blood. The blood carries the nutrients to all the cells of our bodies.

Inside the cells, some nutrients are burned and their energy is extracted and used to supply heat and work that is required by the cells. The rest of the nutrients are utilized in building and repairing body cells. When carbohydrates and proteins are not needed, they are converted to fat molecules and stored as fat. Excess vitamins and minerals are excreted from our bodies via the kidneys.

Our bodies are also resourceful. We have mechanisms developed in a way that allow us to re-synthesize new molecules, and convert one type of molecule into another. This allows our bodies to acquire adequate nourishment from different foods. For example, we can transform amino acids into fat or glucose, and our body cells are able to switch their source of fuel between sugar (glucose) and fat, depending on which fuel is more convenient under given circumstances. But there are some limitations to this. Amino acids and therefore proteins cannot be made from carbohydrate or fat because carbohydrates and fats do not have nitrogen atoms in their molecular construction. Nor can our bodies synthesize vitamins and minerals from organic molecules. However, all three major nutrients, proteins, fats, and carbohydrates, can be used interchangeably in our bodies as fuel because all three major nutrients contain carbon that is readily burned.

Our bodies know how to digest the food, absorb it, automatically decide what nutrients to burn first, what nutrients to convert to fat and store for later use, and when to utilize stored fat for energy. We have no control over any of our bodies' innate physiological functions, nor can we make our bodies burn fat by rationing our food intake. There are many neurochemicals, endorphins and hormones that regulate and control our metabolic activities automatically and shift the body from burning glucose to burning fat according to our physiological needs.

Chapter 3

Physiological Processes

Homeostasis

The human body is a collection of complex mechanisms with many functions and parts. All the different parts of the body fit together ever so intricately into a total, thinking, sensing, functioning human being who can live almost automatically. About one hundred trillion cells make up the human body. Each cell is a living unit, capable of performing chemical and biological functions that the body as a whole depends upon to maintain life and well-being.

The most important requirement for the cells of our bodies is the maintenance of a constant composition of the bodily fluids that bathe the cells. These fluids must be maintained and controlled at a specific set level at all times. The maintenance of a constant condition around the cells is called *homeostasis.*

A healthy body can maintain constant conditions because every organ plays its role in the control of one or more of the fluid constituents. For instance, the circulatory system, composed of the heart and blood vessels, transports blood throughout the body. All the dissolved substances diffuse back and forth between the blood and the fluids that surround the cells. The circulatory system keeps the internal fluids of all the parts of the body constantly mixed. The respiratory system transfers oxygen from the air to the blood. Then oxygen is transported to the tissue fluid surrounding the cells in order to maintain the oxygen levels required for the metabolic activities of those cells. Carbon dioxide is diffused from the tissue fluid into the blood, and is removed through the lungs. The digestive system breaks down food nutrients which are then absorbed into the bloodstream and transported to where they can be used by the cells. The endocrine glands and the liver convert the nutrients absorbed from the gastrointestinal tract into substances that can be used by the cells. The kidneys remove the remains of the nutrients after the cells have used their energy. The sensory organs of touch, hearing, smelling, tasting, and sight protect the body from danger. They also regulate body temperature, search for and select food. All parts of the body work together to create a stable and ideal environment, necessary for the survival of the being as a whole. Homeostasis is not static. The body constantly adjusts its regulatory mechanisms to cause internal changes in order to maintain constant internal conditions in the face of the changing external environment.

The Body Metabolism

The term metabolism simply refers to the chemical reactions that occur in the living body. These reactions occur inside the individual cells and tissues. Metabolic reactions provide us with energy so we can perform our activities and build new structures. It is

Chapter 3

because of the metabolic process that our cells grow larger and increase in number. Thus our body metabolism is not only for energy needs but also for growth, repair of damage to our cells, and the production of new cells.

Metabolic reactions are inherent functions of every cell. However, the rate of metabolism is controlled by the action of hormones secreted by the endocrine system. The endocrine system is made up of many glands in various locations in the body. Each gland secretes minute quantities of hormones into the bloodstream. The endocrine system is controlled by the hormones produced by the cells in the hypothalamus (a part of the brain which will be discussed in the next section). A very delicate vascular system interconnects the hypothalamus with the pituitary gland (an important endocrine center), so the hypothalamus greatly influences the secretions of pituitary hormones. Most pituitary hormones control the secretions of other endocrine glands.

Endorphins are biochemicals released during the passage of sensory messages through the nerves. There are many different substances and biochemicals involved in the transmitting of various sensory messages through the nerve cells. Endorphins are specific neurochemicals that seem to take away sensations of pain and cause elation and happy feelings.

Neurochemicals work in close concert with the endocrine system and together they control and regulate all body functions. They speed up or slow down our metabolism, regulate water balance and electrolyte balance (sodium and potassium balance) and maintain homeostasis. They induce changes so we can cope with stressful situations. They control reproduction, promote growth and development, and control our internal body functions that are outside the realm of our consciousness and voluntary control. These functions include sweating, digestion, and blood circulation. The actions of the autonomic nervous system are involuntary in contrast to the somatic nervous system which controls the voluntary actions of the skeletal muscles.

The Hypothalamus

It is important to learn about the hypothalamus because it contains the centers for regulating all internal body functions, including thirst, hunger, taste, smell, feeding, and satiety. It has areas that control the speed of food digestion and absorption, the rate of blood flow, and the regulation of body temperature. It also controls the thyroid gland and the metabolic rate. Most importantly, the centers for excitement, rage, and other emotions are also located here. This part of the brain has a direct link to the conscious thinking and memory part of our brain. The hypothalamus seems to hold the key to our physical and emotional well-being. Any disturbance in this part of the brain results in metabolic (weight) disturbances (remember our rat from Chapter 1) and emotional upheaval.

All sensory messages from the tongue, the liver, the stomach, and the intestines terminate in the same location in the hypothalamus. This area is known as the nucleus of the solitary tract. This nucleus processes information about nutrients that have been eaten and absorbed. Other nutrient related information from various parts of the body are also monitored in the hypothalamus such as the levels of sugar and carbon dioxide in the blood. All of the self-regulatory centers that control internal automatic functions are controlled by the hypothalamus.

Emotions and Behavior

All sensory feelings from all parts of our bodies travel to our brain through a network of nerve pathways and extended axons. Messages from the brain travel back through nerve pathways reaching every organ, muscle, and tissue. Nerve cells generate electrochemical impulses that travel from sensory organs to the brain through the nerve pathways. These biochemically generated impulses travel very much like electric currents along the nerve and are transferred from one nerve cell to another at the nerve endings. At the nerve endings, nerve fibers branch out to much finer tentacles called dendrites.

Sensory messages traveling from all parts of the body to the brain, terminate in a specific location at the base of the brain. Each of these locations is designed to decode the information that it receives. These locations are interconnected with each other to form a combined network of centers called the limbic system. Behavioral patterns that are aimed at survival of the individual such as attack, searching for food, and those conducive to perpetuation of the species, such as sociosexual activities are also located in the base of the brain within the limbic system. In experimental animals, stimulating specific locations of the limbic system brings about certain behaviors. Stimulation in one area brings about anger and rage in an otherwise docile animal. Stimulation in another area causes tameness and placidity. Stimulation in yet another area called the amygdala, induces sexual behavior and copulatory movements. Stimulation of certain lesions in the amygdala can change sexual behavior and the animal even attempts to mate with different species.

All the various centers in the limbic system are responsible for spontaneous internal responses, preparing the body systems to respond to the emotional state of the person. For example, the tensing of the skeletal muscles and increased heart rate and breathing occur in anticipation of an attack or during anger. There are specific centers in the brain for every sensation that we experience and scientists are still mapping the locations of various centers responsible for each behavior. However, one cannot speak of an emotional center. Each group of neurons becomes connected with each other group of neurons in a specific way, and specific groups of neurons are linked with continual traffic via the hypothalamus between the cerebral cortex, and the limbic system, all contributing to setting an emotional state. This complex, interacting network is associated with emotions. Emotions encompass feelings and moods such as anger, fear, and happiness. The various neurochemicals and endorphins released during brain activities modulate the moods and emotions which we experience.

Executing complex behavior such as mating or attacking requires interaction between almost all of the

sensory organs and the outside world. For complex reactions, our brain brings into play the higher cortical
mechanisms that control thought process to manifest
behaviors necessary to deal with the outside world so
that appropriate behavior is undertaken. Our cerebral
cortex provides the mechanisms needed for implemen-
tation of the required muscular movements, or a plan
to approach or avoid the adversary, or to participate in
a sexual activity, or display emotional expression.

Noticeable physical changes become reflected in our
expressions, for example: laughing, crying, smiling, and
blushing. These external displays appear in response to
internal manifestations of emotions, causing changing
of facial expressions, such as the tightening up of skeletal muscles in preparedness for an attack or flight.

Humans learn to consciously suppress or recall some
programmed expressions. For example, a smile is the
universal human expression that appears on the face
reflecting happiness and contentment. But it can also
be produced consciously when posing for a camera.
Smiling is apparently programmed in the cortex and
can be called upon by the limbic system. Smiling is a
facial expression which automatically appears on the
face of a newborn baby. The smile could not have been
learned or imitated because the same smiling expression appears on the face of a newborn blind baby as
well.

In humans the involvement of the cortex is addi-
tionally important for the conscious awareness of emotion. The cortex, which involves thought, memory, and
learning, further reinforces, modifies, or suppresses behavior patterns. The consequential actions of emotional

behavior are guided by planning, strategy, and judgment based on understanding and learning.

Learning

Learning is the ability to acquire knowledge through experience or instructions, or both. Scientists believe that reward and punishment are integral parts of learning. Learning results from detecting a sensory stimuli and relating it to a similar memory of a stimuli, through a complex neuronal network that produces changes in the way we perceive, act, and feel. Learning establishes new pathways and connections through the brain circuitry, resulting in more dendrites and the production of more endorphins. There are several types of learning which are dependent on the organism's interaction with the environment.

When a particular experience results in punishment, an animal will shy away and avoid repeating that experience. When an experience results in a reward, an animal will seek that experience. This type of learning is referred to as conditional learning.

The mechanism of learning is complex and there are many neurochemicals involved in the process. Endorphins have an important role in the process of reinforcement because they suppress pain and elevate mood.

In 1954, James Olds conducted an experiment on the parts of the brain which were thought to be learning centers. He thought that electrical stimulation of these areas might increase arousal and facilitate learning. Along with his assistant Peter Milner, he placed electrodes into the brain of a rat and by accident they missed their target. The electrodes were instead placed in the pleasure center in the hypothalamus. Olds describes what happened:

> I applied a brief train of 60-cycle-wave of electrical current into the electrode whenever the animal entered one corner of the enclosure. The animal did not stay away from the corner but rather came back quickly after a brief sortie which followed the first stimulation and came back even more quickly after a brief sortie which followed the second stimulation. By the time the third electrical stimulation had been applied the animal seemed indubitably to be coming back for more (Olds, J., Commentary, 1973 p. 81).

Olds and Milner were very intrigued with this result. They implanted electrodes in the brains of several rats and allowed the animals to administer their own stimulation, by pressing a lever. Their study reported that the animals administered self-stimulations at rates exceeding seven hundred stimulations per hour. In subsequent studies where better levers were devised, rats administered self-stimulations at rates exceeding several thousand per hour. It is clear that electrical stimulation of certain parts of the brain can reinforce behavior.

How Does Brain Stimulation Reinforce Behavior?

Many scientists believe that electrical stimulation of the brain activates the same system that is activated by natural reinforcers, such as eating, drinking, or sexual activities. In scientific experiments when the tip of an electrode is placed in a specific location in the brain and the current is turned on, depending on the location of the electrode, an animal would engage in a species-typical behavior such as eating, drinking, copulating, or shredding nesting material. Electrical stimulation of certain other locations can cause aversive effects, not reinforcing ones. When an electrode is planted in a location that controls aversive behaviors such as fear, pain, or anger, the animal will consider the stimulation as punishment and avoid pushing the lever to administer self-stimulations.

A special technique discovered in 1962 called the Histofluorescence method can precisely locate certain kinds of neurotransmitter substances in brain tissue. When brain tissue is exposed to dry formaldehyde gas, certain neurons fluoresce bright yellow under an ultraviolet light. This method allowed scientists to trace the various locations of dopaminergic (meaning neurons that work with the neurochemical dopamine. "*Ergic*" from Greek means work) and other endorphin releasing neurons in the brain. This means that scientists were able to precisely locate the sites of the electrodes, and could be certain about which parts of the brain were being stimulated.

The nervous system, composed of the brain, the spinal cord and all sensory neurons in various sensory organs, controls all the physiological processes of the body. The brain has an elaborate system to gather and process all the information it needs in order to govern and control all bodily functions in an organized and harmonious manner.

Sensory organs, together with various neurons throughout our bodies gather information about the internal and the external environment and convey it to the brain where it is decoded and analysed. Consequently the brain initiates a reaction in response to the stimuli it receives and transmits it to the muscles or organs. All messages in the nervous system are transmitted in the form of electrochemical impulses, initiating an appropriate reaction. All sensory experiences, together with the body's reaction to the stimuli, are then stored in memory to be referred to later when the body encounters similar circumstances.

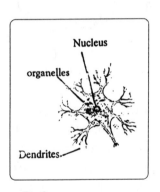

Fig. 2   Nerve Cell

Nerve cells, although microscopic in structure, have long extensions called axons. The longest axons can extend up to two meters long reaching from the tip of the toes to a specific center in the brain (depending on one's height). Nerve fibers are arranged in bundles, much like telephone lines, and carry electrochemical impulses generated by sensory stimuli, conveying information from the sensory organs to the brain and returning directives from the brain to various muscles, organs, and glands.

Nerve cells have a cell body that contains a nucleus and other organelles as shown in Fig. 2. Several tentacles, called dendrites, project from the cell body and terminate in fine branches increasing the surface area of the cell as in Fig. 3. Dendrites are located at the receiving end of a nerve cell.

Each nerve cell also has a single tubular fibre which carries signals away from the cell, called the axon. Axons also branch out into fine tubules and terminate in

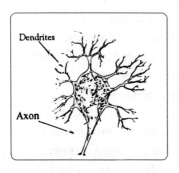

Fig.3   Dendrites

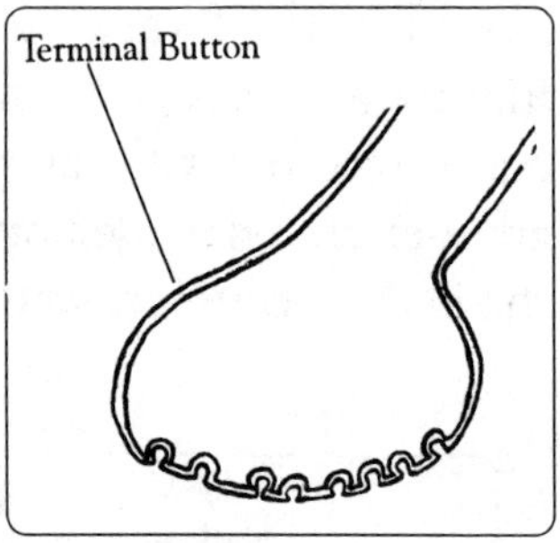

Fig.4   Terminal Button

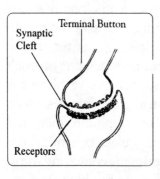

Fig. 5 Synaptic Cleft

button-like endings, called terminal buttons as in Fig 4. The terminal button of one nerve and the dendritic end of another nerve come close together and form a cleavage. This small cleavage between these two surfaces (a terminal button and dendrites) is called the synaptic cleft as in Fig. 5 . Within the synaptic cleft sensory stimuli is transferred from one nerve ending to another. This is where endorphins and neurochemicals are released.

Sensory organs have specific nervous tissues that are able to detect different environmental stimuli. For example the retina of the eye senses light and differentiates the various wave lengths of red, yellow, and green enabling us to see in color. Neurons in the ear recognize repetitive vibrations of sound. The taste buds recognize the molecular structure of foods we eat. Sensory nerve endings in the skin sense touch, pressure, temperature, movement, and vibrations.

When a sensory neuron of the ear recognizes a sound stimulus, or the neurons in the retina of the eye detect light waves, or a pin prick triggers a neuron in the skin, the sensation takes the form of a pattern of electric charges that are transferred along the axon to the brain cells, or another neighboring nerve cell. As the charges transfer from one cell to another at the synaptic cleft, neurochemicals are released. These neurochemicals change the polarization of the receptors which are found in the synaptic cleft, and together with the type of the receptor they polarize, cause either an *excitatory* or *inhibitory* result. Excitatory effects allow sensory messages to pass through the synaptic junctions where the neurochemicals are released. Inhibitory effects inhibit or block the sensory messages from passing through. This simple action of allowing or blocking sensory messages from reaching the brain cells, effectively places neurochemicals in control of the body's reactionary mechanisms and makes the work of the brain very easy. (In a sense this "allowing" or "blocking" of messages is similar to the binary system used by computers). It is as simple as this, if the messages are blocked from reaching the brain, the brain cannot receive sensory information and therefore we do not react to the sensation initiated in a sensory organ. This is how pain killing medications work. The painkillers block messages of pain detected by pain sensing neurons from reaching the center for pain in the hypothalamus.

Because transmitter substances have excitatory and inhibitory effects, one might expect there to be two transmitter substances, excitatory and inhibitory. There are actually many different neurotransmitter substances. Although some do appear to be exclusively excitatory or inhibitory, others can produce either excitatory or inhibitory effects depending on the nature of the synaptic receptors they activate.

The nervous system contains a variety of transmitter substances and they interact with specific nerve receptors. Receptors are very complex. They contain sites that can recognize two or more different transmitter substances. They also contain binding sites that can be activated or blocked. Once a transmitter substance is released, it will stimulate, or inhibit stimulation of the receptor in the synaptic cleft. Scientists have discovered many drugs that act on receptors. Some drugs bind with the receptors mimicking the effects of transmitter substances, while others activate the receptors. One type of drugs occupy the receptors without activating them and prevent transmitter substances from activating them, these types of drugs are called receptor blockers. Most painkilling drugs directly block sensations of pain from reaching the brain by blocking the transfer of electrochemical currents at the synaptic cleft.

There are enzymes present in the synaptic cleft

which can destroy excess neurotransmitter substances. Alternately transmitter substances can be absorbed back into the nerve cells from where they were released. Drugs sometimes interfere in the destruction or the reabsorption of the transmitter substances, permitting these molecules to remain active in the synaptic cleft for longer periods of time. For example, amphetamine and cocaine prevent the reabsorption of norepinephrine and dopamine, prolonging the effects of dopamine which remain active for a longer period, giving the cocaine user prolonged feelings of euphoria.

There are several kinds of neurochemicals, and we are able to release these chemicals naturally as a result of our various sensory activities. The combination and the amounts of these neurochemicals released during our day to day activities set our moods and determine our emotional state. These chemicals allow us to experience a wide range of emotional feelings. Our moods can vary from feelings of elation to feelings of sadness and depression. As an example, when we release dopamine, it suppresses pain by inhibiting the transmission of the pain message from the neuron to the centers for pain and anxiety and we feel good. When we do not release sufficient dopamine, we feel depressed.

Drugs and alcohol also affect our mood. For example, when we drink alcoholic beverages, our inhibitions become suppressed in two ways. First, the alcohol in the drink temporarily blocks aversive sensations from reaching the centers for anxiety in the brain, therefore we appear and feel more relaxed. Also alcohol excites dopaminergic neurons triggering the release of dopamine. It is this combination of the effects of alcohol and the extra dopamine in the system that gives the user an artificial high.

A person's mood is determined according to the amounts of neurochemicals present in the brain and according to the types of these neurochemicals. The physiological processes of the brain are designed so that living organisms are able to learn from their own experiences and situations. This ability to learn from experience by associating it with the resulting pleasure or pain allows the organism to choose or avoid certain experiences. Therefore organisms will be able to "learn" and innately know to pursue the activities that will make them feel good. Neurochemicals and endorphins released during all our actions, produce pleasant or unpleasant feelings which condition us to behave in a manner most conducive to survival and enhancement of our lot in life.

Other substances that can influence our neurochemical and endorphin producing mechanisms have been found in nature, or prepared in laboratories. Some of these substances, used wisely, can help alleviate and cure many mental disturbances, but in the hands of the naivé and ill-informed, these drugs are often abused and become dangerous and detrimental to the health and the well-being of their users.

Recommended reading: L. Sherwood 1989, Human Physiology, West Publishing Company, St Paul MN.

Chapter 4

Endorphins

The Discovery Of Endorphins

Nature has intended for us to experience happy feelings, so that we become hooked on living, and overcome our weak moments and sad feelings, go on living and seeking the activities that promote the experiences that make us feel happy. Our well-being is directly linked to all life-enriching activities. We have built-in mechanisms that know how to pull us out of sad moments and restore our mood.

Everyone knows what it is like to be happy and sad. We also know that there are different levels to these feelings. Sometimes we feel really good about ourselves, we are at the top of the world and nothing can shake us. Other times we feel that the earth should open up and swallow us quietly, and we would not put up a fight. But soon these feelings go away once we start to go on about our daily business and immerse ourselves in the tasks and activities we must accomplish.

Of course there are various chemical compounds that we might get a prescription for or we may even buy on street corners that can improve our moods and make us feel better. But we also know that taking chemicals to elevate our mood is not the answer because once we start taking chemical substances we will need to keep taking them, becoming dependent on them, and we will not be able to feel good without them. For the same reason, some people resort to food, tobacco, or alcohol to make them feel better. Most people know how to get out of their slump without resorting to any chemicals or food to make them feel good about themselves. Living organisms do not need to take any chemicals to help them elevate their mood. All living organisms including human beings are able to manufacture their own mood changing chemicals naturally. When our sensory organs detect a change in our environment, the sensation causes an electrochemical current to flow through our nerves and reach the brain, releasing specific neurochemicals in the process.

In 1953, Sir Henry Dale, the renowned physiologist, originated the idea that all neurons release the same biochemical at all their nerve endings. This idea gained widespread support after it was proved in a laboratory that mammalian spinal motoneurons release a substance called acetylcholine. Later it was discovered that acetylcholine belongs to a group of substances that can alter mood by causing the individual to feel happier. Dopamine, norepinephrine, serotonin, histamine, and enkephalin are all substances synthesized in the nerve cells and their quantities in the body reflect and regulate our mood and emotional state. These neurochemicals are also called endorphins. They are mood-elevating, happiness-causing molecules, synthesized and released in the body during neuronal activity when sensory messages are transferred from one nerve cell to another at the nerve endings.

Chapter 4

People have known for a long time that there is a relationship between the mood of a person and certain chemicals, and that there is a relationship between mood changing chemicals and behavior. In 1563 the Portuguese physician Garcia d'Orta observed that the use of opium diminished sexual activity and even caused impotence (Changeux, 1985). Drugs that block the effects of opiates, such as naloxone, provoke erection in men and monkeys. The administration of opiates diminishes the number of copulations and the percentage of successful mountings in the male hamster. After orgasm, the blood level of endorphin-like peptides increases markedly in the hamster by at least four times after five ejaculations (Murphy, Bowie, & Pert 1979). This perhaps explains why our sexual appetite diminishes after orgasm.

During the last few decades scientists were able to verify that many of these mood changing chemicals are naturally produced in the body. It also became clear that these mood changing chemicals are the basis for our ability to learn and enjoy our lives. The mechanisms by which the body produces these chemicals give us the ability to develop an internal intelligence that promotes and advances the living organism to choose the activities necessary for life. The neurochemicals that are released as a result of the sensory messages transferred in the nerve cells, promote and compel the organism to undertake the activities essential to the business of living.

Imagine billions of neurons, from all of our senses converging at the brain, carrying a wealth of information from every corner of the body. Meissner's corpuscles are sensory nerves sensing touch which are found in the hairless parts of the body. The density of these corpuscles in the palm of the hand and the sole of the foot is about nine thousand neurons per square inch. There are more than a billion other sensory neurons causing wave upon wave of sensation to reach the brain cells from all over the body. Sensations of touch, smell, taste, balance, sound, and vision reach the brain at split second intervals. They excite various locations in the brain and inform us of who we are, what we are doing, and what is happening around us. According to the information we receive, we learn how to deal with the various sensations. We learn to use the information that we receive to avoid pain now, and in the future.

Imagine billions of sensory messages traveling up and down the nerve pathways, changing the positive and the negative charges on the surface of the nerve membrane. These activities are manufacturing mood-elevating substances, which make us feel good.

Mood-Elevating Drugs and Addiction

All mood-elevating drugs excite certain neuronal cells in the brain (dopaminergic neurons), artificially increasing the release of dopamine in the body. This results in an artificially induced elated feeling. Addiction is the result of neurons developing tolerance to repeated excitatory stimuli caused by the drug, and a person using a drug requires increasingly larger doses of the drug to attain the same feeling of elation. If drug users do not keep increasing the doses of the drug they have developed a tolerance to, they will experience withdrawal symptoms. Withdrawal symptoms produce opposite effects to those caused by the drug. For example, where heroin produces euphoria, withdrawal symptoms cause an anxious feeling, dysphoria. Heroin produces relaxation, and withdrawal causes agitation. Heroin causes constipation and withdrawal causes diarrhoea and cramps (Carlson, 1990).

When people start taking substances that artificially trigger the production of endorphins in their bodies, and their neurons become desensitized to sensory stimuli (in other words, they become addicted to a certain drug), they render themselves unable to receive pleasure by employing their senses. Desensitized neurons cannot possibly become excited by sensory stimuli and produce the neurochemicals that are required to restore our mood. Therefore drug users cannot manufacture their own mood elevating neurochemicals naturally by employing their senses, and they must depend on drugs to produce the neurochemicals that they need to restore their mood. They become preoccupied with satisfying their ever-increasing need to get more drugs to prevent the anxious misery of withdrawal symptoms. (Over time, drug use creates a vicious cycle: as abusers take more and more of a drug, their tolerance for that drug increases, demanding them to take even more, which increases their tolerance even more, and so on.) They neglect all other aspects of their lives that could give them the means for releasing endorphins naturally. To kick the drug habit, an addict must endure the suffering and withdrawal symptoms, and abstain from using drugs to allow time to heal and re-sensitize the neurons that were desensitized by the drugs. They must abstain from the drug until their dopaminergic neurons resume the ability to produce neurochemicals in response to sensory stimuli. When they start producing their own dopamine without taking drugs, the urge to take drugs will subside.

Drug addicts often develop psychotic behaviors, which include mood disturbances, hallucinations, delusions of persecution, and repetitive behavior. These behaviors closely resemble the behavior of paranoid schizophrenia. After drug users kick their habit, their psychotic reactions subside. However, exposure to these drugs produces long term changes in their brain, and the psychotic reactions will resurface when reformed drug users later encounter the drug they were addicted to, even after several years of abstinence from it (Sato, Chen, Akiyama & Otsuki, 1983; Sato, 1986). Perhaps this explains why people who quit smoking become extremely agitated and angry when they are subjected to nicotine in second hand smoke.

Caffeine

Caffeine is a stimulant. It has addictive effects and large doses of caffeine can become harmful to health. However, it is relatively harmless in non-pregnant adults and when taken in small doses. The effects of caffeine differ from individual to individual, depending on the size of the person, the amount of caffeine consumed over a period of time, and the extent to which the user has developed a tolerance to it. Caffeine can raise the blood pressure, blood cholesterol levels, and pulse. It also can cause irregular heart beats (Leonard, Watson & Mohs 1987). Caffeine stimulates the digestive tract and peristalsis, promoting bowel evacuation. Its wakening effects are well known. The wakening effect of caffeine is not all that clear, since caffeine increases brain serotonin concentrations, which is generally associated with relaxation and placidity (Leonard, Watson & Mohs, 1988).

Caffeine is found in plants including coffee beans, tea leaves, and cocoa beans. Caffeine is added to soft drinks, some pain relievers, and most over-the-counter weight-control aids. It is found in chocolates and all beverages that contain chocolate. The FDA stipulates that all products containing caffeine must specify on the label the amount of caffeine added to the package but does not require reporting the caffeine content of products having naturally-occurring caffeine. For example, a chocolate bar contains cocoa, but the package does not report the amount of caffeine in that candy bar. You must read the labels of the foods you purchase to find out what you are consuming! You must also acquaint yourself with the products that contain caffeine, naturally or artificially.

Withdrawal from coffee often causes severe headaches. When one experiences a severe headache after being under an anaesthetic, the headache is often caused by caffeine withdrawal rather than the anaesthetic. As soon as they are able to drink coffee the headache subsides.

Besides its wakening effects, caffeine also has other physiological and psychological effects. It can improve endurance when taken in moderate doses, about 2 milligrams per pound of body weight or two to three cups one hour before exercise (Costill, Dalsky & Fink, 1978). Caffeine facilitates the utilization of fatty-acids as an energy source, thus helping to spare the use of muscle glycogen for the later stages of prolonged aerobic exercise. Caffeine can make exercising seem easier, but one does not need caffeine to help release fatty acids before exercise. Stretching and warm up exercises also facilitate the release of free fatty acids, making exercising easier and muscles more flexible and less susceptible to injury, while caffeine does not.

Nicotine

Nicotine stimulates the acetylcholine receptors and dopaminergic neurons, causing acetylcholine and dopamine to be released in the brain (Damsma, Day & Fibiger, 1989). Although nicotine is a milder drug than most other dopaminergic stimulants, many people who try it go on to become addicts.

Nicotine addiction should not be underestimated; the combination of nicotine and other substances in tobacco are carcinogenic, and smoking often leads to cancer of the mouth, throat and lungs. Cigarette smoking coats the lining of the air-sacs, *alveoli,* in the lungs, restricting the passage of oxygen through the lining of the lungs to the blood. Nicotine also causes constriction of the blood vessels, raising the blood pressure and limiting blood supplies to many parts of the body including the heart muscle. This can eventually lead to heart attack.

Smoking has some connections to eating, appetite, and weight control. Smoking cigarettes does ease feelings of hunger. When smokers feel hungry, they can suppress it by smoking instead of eating. Such behavior ignores body signals and retards innate mechanisms of our bodies that control eating. (Refer to Chapter 6, Sensory Organs and The Mechanisms That Control Eating). Nicotine and other chemicals in cigarettes specifically tar, act as a local anaesthetic and numb the taste buds so smokers cannot properly taste the foods they eat. This further renders smokers insensitive to what they eat.

Smokers tend to gain weight when they give up smoking (Carney & Goldberg, 1984). Weight gain is a major concern for people who are contemplating quitting smoking. Cigarette smokers should not worry about the slight weight gain anticipated upon quitting the habit. Once they give it up and develop their lungs and cardiovascular system, training their muscles to draw their energy 100 percent from fat, the initial weight gain from quitting smoking will soon disappear. (Refer to Chapter 7, Lean Mean Fat Burning Machine)

Alcohol

Alcohol abuse is a menace to society. A large percentage of death, injuries, and illnesses are alcohol related. Women drinking alcohol during pregnancy give birth to babies with malformed brains and brain damage, resulting in numerous defective physical and mental characteristics more commonly known as Fetal Alcohol Syndrome. The leading cause of mental retardation in the western world today is alcohol consumption by pregnant women (Abel & Sokol, 1986).

A small dose of alcohol produces mild euphoria, be-

cause it reduces anxiety. Larger doses produce sedation and a lack of coordination. It is believed that alcohol produces both positive and negative reinforcement. The antianxiety effects of alcohol, are negative
reinforcers, causing a person to drink when confronted
with difficult and anxious moments. The positive reinforcing aspect of alcohol is that it stimulates
dopaminergic neurons to release dopamine and gives
the user a euphoric feeling. Alcohol increases the firing of the dopaminergic neurons, releasing dopamine
in the brain (Gessa, Muntoni, Collu, Vargiu & Mereu,
1985).

Alcohol is highly addictive. Its withdrawal effects
are dangerous and can be fatal. Convulsions caused by
alcohol withdrawal (*Delirium tremens*) are considered
a medical emergency, and are treated with barbiturates.
Barbiturates have effects similar to those of alcohol and
the combination of barbiturates and alcohol intensi-
fies the sedation effects of these drugs resulting in an
overdose of dopamine in the body. Marilyn Monroe is
believed to have died mixing alcohol and barbiturates.

Alcohol arises naturally from carbohydrates when
certain microorganisms metabolize them in the absence
of oxygen. The process is more commonly known as
fermentation. If a wine making apparatus is not air tight
then fermentation occurs in the presence of oxygen
and the carbohydrates will be converted into vinegar
instead of wine. Fermenting plants rich in carbohydrates
such as grapes, apples, potatoes, and many other fruits
and vegetables, and changing their juices to wine or
spirits has been practiced by many civilizations for more
than 5,000 years. The euphoric aspects of alcoholic

beverages have encouraged many people to use them in various ceremonies and celebrations.

Alcohol is a fat solvent and it destroys the cell membranes it comes in contact with. When ingested it does not have to be digested. It is absorbed directly into the bloodstream and within one minute of consumption, alcohol reaches the brain. It first impairs judgment and reasoning, then effects motor control, causing loss of balance, and eventually it effects the breathing and heart action causing death. The first drink a person takes often sets the scene for bizarre behavior if the user keeps drinking more than half an ounce of liquor per hour, which is the rate at which the liver can metabolize alcohol. If the person drinks at a faster rate than one shot per hour, blood alcohol levels rise, and alcohol molecules circulate in the blood, reaching all parts of the body where they irritate and damage the cells.

Liver cells are the only cells that can break down alcohol molecules and they must work extra hard to produce the special enzymes which accomplish this. When liver cells are busy breaking down alcohol molecules, they are not able to carry out their many other important functions. The liver is the intermediary metabolism and storage center for most of the nutrients required by our bodies. It splits fats and proteins into smaller substances so our cells can use them for energy. It forms products needed for blood clotting, for transporting fat, for immunity to infection, and for many other purposes. The liver also stores large quantities of fat, carbohydrates, and proteins, then releases these nutrients when the tissues need them. An animal will die without a liver within a few hours. Long term abuse of alcohol eventually destroys liver cells, causing cirrhosis of the liver. A malfunctioning liver will cause all other body systems to malfunction as well, because all energy supplies are processed by the liver. Metabolic disturbances will eventually cause a general system failure, and irreversible damage to many organs and systems of the body including the brain, leading to chronic illnesses and eventual death.

Alcohol molecules are broken down into smaller molecules and used for energy. Whatever is not burned as energy accumulates in the liver and is converted to fat.

The Reinforcing Mechanisms Of The Body

The reinforcing mechanisms of our bodies are designed to make us pursue the activities that give us pleasure, so we may learn to respond to activities that improve our lives and our well-being. Unfortunately there are many chemicals available to us (manufactured in laboratories or found naturally in various plants), that can also stimulate our reinforcing mechanisms. We can easily become addicted to them. Once we become addicted to these chemicals we no longer can use our natural and inherent reinforcement mechanisms which teach us to do what enhances our lives. We instead pursue drug use to make us feel good, and become unable to benefit from our innate reinforcing mechanisms to lead a healthy life.

Olds and Milner's experiment with a rat who came back to receive more electrical charges through the rods planted in its hypothalamus (Chapter 3), led to considerable progress in understanding the mechanisms of reinforcement. Many more studies by various scientists led to the understanding that all substances that reinforce behavior by exciting dopaminergic neurons can lead to addiction. These substances have an excitatory effect on various centers of the brain where dopaminergic neurons are found. The excitation of dopaminergic neurons releases dopamine which changes the mood of the person taking these drugs, giving the user an artificial feeling of elation.

Caffeine, nicotine, alcohol, and the harder drugs such as marijuana, cocaine, heroin, have all been found to stimulate dopaminergic neurons in the hypothalamus and release dopamine. The primary reason for addiction is the reinforcing effect of these substances. An addict stays addicted not because of a fear of the unpleasant symptoms these drugs produce when an addict is trying to quit, but rather because of their reinforcing euphoric effects.

All habit forming drugs are interrelated in that they all stimulate the dopaminergic neurons and release dopamine. When a person is addicted to several substances, the use of one drug could potentially trigger the desire to use all the other drugs that person is addicted to (like "when I drink I've got to smoke"). This contributes to relapse when the user of the drug is attempting to abstain from one of the drugs that he or she is addicted to. For example, people who are attempting to quit smoking will more likely succeed if they also abstain from drinking coffee as well. For the same reason, cigarette smoking could cause an alcohol abstainer to relapse. The excitation of dopaminergic neurons by one chemical triggers the release of dopamine and awakens the desire for all the other chemicals that the person is addicted to. Many addiction treatment centers and AA chapters are beginning to realize the value of abstinence from all co-addictions when attempting to abstain from alcohol or more severe drugs. Giving up smoking and coffee along with alcohol or harder drugs, can improve the success rates of their clients.

Experiments on animals show that if self-administered cocaine or heroin is stopped through non-reinforcement, an injection of a drug that stimulates dopaminergic neurons can reinstate the addictive habit. Similarly, smoking primes the dopaminergic receptors and contribute to relapse in people who are trying to abstain from taking other harder drugs. Because nicotine excites dopaminergic neurons, smoking could potentially make it more difficult for an alcohol or heroin user to abstain from their addictions (Wise, 1990).

Endorphins Control Eating & Learning Behaviors

Eating and learning are closely associated in that they both involve recording in our memories the sensory experiences which we encounter. Later when we encounter similar circumstances, we rely on previous experiences to recognize and formulate a plan of action to deal with new similar situations. During eating we learn about the taste, texture, and smell of the foods that we eat, and how the food satisfies our hunger. When we later encounter a need for the same nutrients, we will automatically crave for the foods we have eaten before.

Complex neuronal processes result in changing the structure of brain cells, establishing new pathways and more dendrites, thus changing the way we perceive and feel. Eating results in conditional learning of the foods we eat. Many experiments have demonstrated that the neurochemical serotonin is released during both learning and eating. Several studies confirm the involvement of serotonin in hunger and satiety and its relation to carbohydrate intake and fat. Serotonin is released in the hypothalamus during eating (Stanley, Shwartz, Hernendase, Leibowitz & Hoebel, 1989). The presence of serotonin in the hypothalamus reduces the desire for carbohydrates but has no effect on the desire for fat in rats (Leibowitz, Weiss, Walsh & Viswanath, 1989). Drugs that reduce or inhibit production of serotonin cause an increase in appetite. (Breisch, Zelman & Hoebel, 1976). Serotonin is an inhibitory chemical. When it is released, it blocks the actions of another excitatory neurochemical called norepinephrine, which has an effect opposite to serotonin. It increases the desire for carbohydrates and initiates hunger.

We know from our experience that when we are busy doing interesting projects, food is the last thing on our minds. We often skip lunch and keep on doing the thing we are enjoying and do not even feel hungry. On the other hand, when we are frustrated and have nothing to do, many of us think about food, especially sweet things. We think about sweet things because they cause the release of serotonin. After we eat a lot of sweets we feel more relaxed and placid, the appetite for sweets diminishes and the levels of serotonin in the brain rise. It is the release of serotonin that makes us feel relaxed and happy, and we do not feel bored or on edge any more. This happy feeling resembles the good feeling you receive after finding the right piece of a jigsaw puzzle or figuring out the solution to a problem: you feel relaxed and more content but still stimulated.

The Neurochemical Serotonin

The neurochemical serotonin is implicated in both eating and learning. Serotonin is derived from the amino acid tryptophan, a protein utilized by the brain cells. Serotonin is also called 5-hydroxytryptamine or 5-HT. Investigators have identified three different types of serotonin, 5-HT_{1A}, 5-HT_{1B}, 5-HT_2. Serotonin plays a key role in the regulation of mood and in the regulation and control of pain. It is strongly implicated in the mechanism of eating, sleeping, and arousal. Serotonergic neurons (*Ergon* is a Greek word for work: Serotonergic neurons are stimulated by the neurochemical serotonin) are involved somehow in the control of dreaming. The drug LSD seems to produce hallucinations by stimulating 5-HT receptors, and thus causes the person taking LSD to dream while awake (Carlson, 1990).

The emotional states we experience are a reflection of what experiences we have gone through. Our feelings stem from events in our lives, and not all is well at times. We often encounter unpleasant experiences, and if unpleasant experiences are persistent, they may lead to depression. The inability to experience pleasure is one of the main symptoms of depression.

low levels of serotonin in their cerebrospinal fluids, which means that serotonergic neurons in their brains were not releasing enough neurochemicals to elevate their mood (Sulser & Sanders-Bush, 1989).

In an experiment, Vogel, Neill, Hagler, and Kors (1990) altered the hypothalamus of rats and decreased the production of serotonin permanently. These rats exhibited symptoms of depression. They showed decreased sexual behaviors, increased irritability, and decreased pleasure-seeking behaviors by displaying a decreased willingness to work for reinforcing brain stimulation. Furthermore, they had lost their taste for sucrose. These rats also had difficulty sleeping.

The body needs these mood elevating chemicals to maintain a cheerful, well-balanced mental state. The body encounters more than enough of its share of wear and tear which is quite traumatic and stressful. We endure a tremendous amount of stress in day to day living. If it was not for the soothing and mood elevating effects of neurochemicals that we release as a result of our sensory experiences, life would be unbearable. Because eating, particularly eating sweets, has a definite role in releasing serotonin, it is important that we do not use eating to elevate our mood, but rather to experience taste, texture and color of foods we eat, and learn how these foods can satisfy our hunger. Learning about our food, also releases serotonin. Instead of eating because we are bored, we can do something new and exciting which also will release the serotonin that will elevate our mood and we will not resort to food.

Living Life and Loving It

The sensations of pleasure and pain have evolved from the basic survival tool of a single neural axis such as that which is found in the earthworm, which also relaxes or shies away from danger. From this simple system, every multicellular creature in the animal kingdom has developed a network of nerve cells and neuronal pathways which automatically govern all bodily functions. In man a mammoth network of nerves evolved that set the patterns which enable us to form a conscious awareness of our emotions. We have learned to store in our memory the actions that cause pain and pleasure, then we remember to shy away from pain and seek pleasure in our future actions, and in the process produce endorphins to make us feel good.

All living organisms who possess a nervous system experience pain and pleasure. All sensory messages that reach the brain are interpreted on these two terms. Experiences that enhance and promote life span, the perpetuation of the species, and the well-being of the individual organism, cause the production of endorphins. These neurochemicals in turn elevate and heighten the enjoyment of life. Experiences that result in pain also cause the body to release endorphins to relieve the pain and make life bearable in the face of adversity. The mechanism of endorphin production is designed to compel the living organism to pursue activities that give it pleasure. The analgesic effect of endorphins allows the animal to continue painful experiences that are essential for its survival. For example, if an animal is wounded during pursuit of its prey, the animal will still continue its attack and still attempt to secure its food supply, despite the injuries sustained. The body produces endogenous morphine-like substances to ease pain.

The amount of endorphin found in our bodies indicates how we are leading our lives. We are often compelled to indulge in the activities that will increase endorphins in our bodies, so we feel good. The good feelings that we experience condition us to pursue a lifestyle that will continue the release of endorphins so we can be happy and content.

Several studies confirm that depression is caused by abnormal levels of endorphins in the body. Low levels of serotonin in the cerebrospinal fluid correlates with attempts of suicide (Traskmann, Asberg, Bertilsson, & Sjostrand, 1981).

Experimental animals with implanted, self-stimulating devices in their reward centers delivered five thousand stimulations an hour, even shunning food when starving in preference of delivering pleasure to themselves. Pleasure seeking is probably the most powerful tool the body has to help the individual cope with adversities and painful experiences.

How Do We Form Habits?

Habits are acts that we have repeated so often, the activity becomes automatic to us. We develop certain habits to meet our repeated needs on a regular basis. Almost all our habits are formed to help our bodies cope with the external factors involved in satisfying an internal sensation.

The autonomic nervous system, along with the hypothalamus, is responsible for the regulation of the body's internal environment. The cognitive part of the brain works in concert with the internal autonomic functions in matters concerning interactions between the internal environment and the external world. For example, the internal autonomic functions signal a need for eating and sensations of hunger, while the cognitive part of the brain recognizes the sensations of hunger and what we must do to satisfy ourselves. Our mechanisms that control eating trigger craving sensations for various foods required to satisfy our need. One step further would be actual eating. When there is no food available, sensations of hunger diminish temporarily only to return later. Our bodies learn to develop regular habits to accommodate our repeated needs depending on how we can interact with the world around us. Our habits are developed to prepare our bodies to meet the regular changes of the universe around us. All life on earth has this ability to prepare itself to meet the demands of its physiological systems (This idea is explained further in Chapter 13 when we discuss Biological Rhythms). For example, when our need to eat becomes satisfied regularly at noon we start to feel hungry then. If we find the time to have a cigarette just after dinner, then we regularly feel the urge to smoke after dinner. The reason these habits become difficult to break is that they satisfy a need in our bodies and the satisfaction of the need produces neurochemicals which make us feel good. There are certain habits that are good for the health and well-being of the person and other habits, which although momentarily satisfy a need in the body, tend to throw strain on the various systems of the body, causing it harm.

For example, the practice of giving a child something sweet to eat when he or she is hurt leads to the development of a desire for sweet things when the child encounters pain. It was clearly demonstrated in an experiment by Leibowitz, Weiss, Walsh, and Viswanath (1989) that eating, especially carbohydrates, increases the release of serotonin in the hypothalamus.

When a person becomes dependent and learns to deal with stress by eating sweets, it is very difficult to break the dependency. To overcome dependency, we should focus on developing habits that will release tension in other ways, like participating in activities that are healthy and rewarding.

The Struggle In Living

We experience life by living it. Our life experiences and the circumstances we have encountered when young will determine how we will perceive ourselves as we grow older. Our perception of ourselves is often formulated according to our abilities and limitations, on our strengths and weaknesses, and how we see ourselves in relation to these issues. We then establish a self-worth by which we can identify ourselves. This "self-worth" is often referred to as our ego.

When a person encounters a situation that might diminish their self-worth and cannot substantiate and validate the cause, the incident will eventually become forgotten. However, its influence will alter the person's relation to all the elements associated with the incident that diminished or belittled their self-worth. Invalidated conflicts from the past can prevent a person from experiencing pleasure. They often make one feel hurt and sad, even if one has forgotten why.

Sigmund Freud, in his lecture, Some Thoughts on Development and Regression Aetiology said,

> It is immediately obvious that the sexual instincts, from beginning to end of their development, work toward obtaining pleasure; The other instinct, the ego-instinct, has the same aim to start with. But under the influence of the instructress Necessity, they soon learn to replace the pleasure principal by a modification of it. For them the task of avoiding unpleasure turns out to be almost as important as that of obtaining pleasure. The ego discovers that it is inevitable for it to renounce immediate satisfaction, to postpone the obtaining of pleasure, to put up with a little unpleasure and to abandon certain sources of pleasure altogether. An ego thus educated becomes 'reasonable'; It no longer lets itself to become governed by the pleasure principle, but obeys the reality principle, which also at bottom seeks to obtain pleasure, but pleasure which is assured through taking account of reality, even though it is pleasure postponed and diminished. The transition from the pleasure principal to the reality principal is one of the most important steps forward in the ego's development." (Freud Translated by Strachey, 1976)

Children or adolescents who are in the process of developing their self-worth and identity, can easily become hurt when forced to give up their pleasures, especially when their joyful moments are snatched away without them understanding why. As children grow up to become adults, they often have to give up certain pleasurable experiences in return for something else that they also value. When we trade off what gives us pleasure in lieu of attaining self-respect or acceptance by our peers and loved ones, our experience will strengthen us emotionally. The process of sacrificing certain pleasures can add to our self-worth. We discover that we can be strong, and can put up with pain and sacrifice. We will think more of ourselves for being patient, understanding, and courageous, and we grow up to become confident, worthy adults, ready to tackle any problem that comes our way. But when our joyful youth and happy experiences are snatched away from us without our consent or understanding why, we can be thrown into the pits of despair. We will feel devastated and lose whatever self-confidence that we had. Perhaps we will grow up confused, feel small, weak, undignified, and experience many other negative feelings which we have encountered in the "pits of despair" that we try to hide. Such feelings and experiences will give their bearers emotional suffering and pain. Their egos become wounded. The emotional suffering might become forgotten in time, but it will constantly prevent them from enjoying their lives as they grow older.

An injured ego is not like a stab wound that might bleed for a while, then form a scab and heal. Nor it is like a broken bone that can be placed in a cast to become as good as new within weeks. Painful wounds to the ego are hidden in the darkest regions of the mind. Hurt feelings become tucked away and are assumed forgotten, yet they remain vivid and intact; they lament incognito. The person suffering from wounds to the ego is often unaware of them. During the process of thought, the brain constantly refers to all past experiences and constantly encounters these painful incidents. Just like a corn on the sole of the foot makes its pain felt every step of the way, so do the memories of emotional pain. As the person encounters any reminder of the painful incidents, unexpected, raw emotions are awakened, stirring painful scenarios of anguish and suffering over and over again.

People suffering from wounds to their ego are often unable to experience pleasure. They constantly involve themselves in activities that will artificially help them forget their emotional pain. They tend to indulge themselves in overeating, or drinking alcohol, or resort to any other means that will artificially stimulate the release of endorphins so they may alleviate their emotional pain and the silent suffering they endure. People with emotional wounds need to heal themselves so they can experience pleasure more readily and not resort to habits that will only cause them more grief.

For emotional wounds to heal, the person must gather enough courage to review past experiences objectively and constructively, re-examine the circumstances and the situation in an attempt to validate the painful incidents, and come to terms with what has happened. They must evaluate the impact of past painful experiences on their present life, and realize that what was done was done and cannot be changed now. Their past experiences can make them wiser and stronger in the present. It is time for them to get on with their lives and rebuild their self-worth with their new found wisdom and strength. The process of healing emotional wounds is not easy. It requires courage, and a willingness to help oneself to grow and become responsible. It is wise to seek counselling and the assistance of a professional who can guide them in the process.

Chapter 5

Sensory Experiences

Human Beings Are Sensory Creatures

Emotional feelings are an intricate part of our being and affect our behavior in every way possible. We find ourselves somewhere between feelings of utter happiness and joy, to feelings of sorrow, fear, anger, or despair, feelings from which we cannot escape. The hallmark of being alive is feeling!

Contrary to our sensory nature, we have been taught and are expected to behave in a way that ignores our feelings and emotions. At a young age we are taught not to cry when feeling sad, to hide our sexuality, to ignore our desires and wishes, and to do what is considered acceptable to others even if it hurts. We have learned to desensitize ourselves to our own feelings. All body mechanisms and functions are based upon sensory messages and feelings, yet we are taught to lead our lives by becoming insensitive to our feelings. In many instances our lack of sensitivity to our own needs has been the cause of many of our physical and emotional problems.

Our understanding of the body's capabilities are limited. Studies of the brain and manifestations of feelings are very complicated. Each individual has a different interpretation of their emotional feelings. In an experiment, sixty university students were surveyed by Bernard Lyman (1989). The average number of different emotions experienced in a day was 31. The smallest number of emotions experienced was 11 and the largest was 86. Students reported experiencing different emotions up to 50 times a day. They also reported having difficulty in keeping an accurate account of their emotions.

The nervous system, together with the neurochemicals released during our activities, governs every aspect of our lives. Every action of the body is coordinated by a nerve impulse which originates in a sensory organ, then travels to the brain where it is decoded. According to that decoding, an appropriate, prompt, and precise response is initiated. The response is transmitted to the part of the body responsible for performing a function that will maintain the homeostatic condition and preserve well-being. The hypothalamus houses many centers for homeostatic functions, each with a distinct location identified by its different protein. For example the protein angiotensin is found in the center for drinking, thirst, and eating. Other proteins are present in the sexual center. The center for hearing has another type of protein. Groups of neurons with their specific chemicals receive messages from various sensory organs in the body. Although the messages arrive at these different specific centers, they travel to the brain in the same manner as electrical charges. But because they reach different parts of the brain, they are decoded differently. For example, sen-

sory nerves arriving in the brain from the nose terminate in the olfactory center in the hypothalamus. Sensory messages that are generated in the eye reach the
optic center. Because of the actions of different proteins, different sensations are perceived. If we were to
switch the bundle of nerves arriving to the hearing
center with that of sight perhaps we could perceive
sound as image, and vice versa. This is of course a weird
way of thinking about sensation, and it is not something we would normally encounter, but rather it is an
example of what might happen if nerve bundles were
switched. Some people have the ability to experience
sound in colorful images, this ability is referred to *synesthesia.*

The nervous system together with the mechanisms
of feelings and emotions are our navigational tools with
which we explore the world around us and the world
within us. To improve our lives and the world we live
in, we must understand ourselves and our behavior,
and why we feel the way we do. By understanding all
the various feelings and emotions that we experience,
we can bring about the changes which we must make
to improve our lot in life. We need to re-sensitize ourselves to our feelings and respond to the calls from
within.

Sensory Experiences Develop Larger Brains

Emotions fluctuate between feelings of utter
happiness and joy to feelings of anger and despair according to the amount of endorphins produced
in the body. This fluctuation is caused by the sensory

experiences the person encounters. Every sensory message causes the body to produce chemical substances that alter and elevate mood, allowing the individual to feel happy. We have learned that by living in a more stimulating environment we feel more content and happy. Many people pursue hobbies because indulging in such activities stimulates them physically or mentally and makes life more enjoyable. By living an active and stimulating lifestyle we encounter new things and different experiences. The more active we are, the more excited our brain cells will become, producing more neurochemicals, making us more happy and content. On the other hand if we do not employ our senses, the level of happiness we experience is not enhanced, and we may even feel sad and depressed.

It has been demonstrated that experiences can affect the very structure of the nervous system, especially if they occur in youth. Rats raised in a stimulating, active environment with several activities to perform, developed larger brains than rats with similar backgrounds who were raised in dull, impoverished environments. Rosenzweig (1984) placed one group of rats in cages containing ladders, tunnels, turning wheels, slides, and toys that the rats could explore and manipulate. They varied the types of toys on a daily basis to maximize experiences and minimize boredom. They placed another group of rats in plain cages in dimly lit, quiet rooms. The brains of the rats raised in the enriched environment had thicker cortices, better capillary blood supply, more glial cells, more protein content, more acetylcholine secreting terminals, and higher endorphin producing capabilities than the brains of rats that lived in impoverished cages. (Glial cells are support cells for neurons. They insulate nerves preventing messages from becoming scrambled, support blood vessels and transport nutrients to nerve cells, and also remove debris and waste materials.)

Each sensory organ has a specific center in the brain that decodes messages arriving from different sensory organs. The more stimulation that a center in the brain receives, the better it will develop. For example a blind person relies heavily upon his senses of touch, smell, and hearing. Probably the centers for touch, smell, and hearing are better developed in a blind person. Perhaps the centers for hearing, smell, and touch are larger in his brain than they would have been if the person had had sight, and perhaps the center for sight in the blind person is not well developed. By the same token, a deaf person, who compensates for his sense of hearing by employing his sense of sight, will have a better developed and larger center of sight in his brain. The body has a rule, anything not used is atrophied and lost, and what is used tends to develop further and grow more.

Turner and Greenough (1985) observed an increase in the size of synapses by 25% per neuron as a result of stimulation of neurons. Greenough and Volkmar (1973) found that rats with enriched upbringing had larger and more complex dendrites. Chang and Greenough (1982) placed an opaque lens on one eye of rats, and allowed visual information from the other eye to reach only the one center for vision in the brain. Then the rats were visually stimulated. The changes in the center of vision were seen only in the vision center receiving messages from the eye that was visually stimulated. These changes indicated better capillary blood supply, more glial cells, more protein content, and more dendrites. These experiments clearly indicate that certain parts of the brain excel independently of the rest of the brain. The acceleration of growth in specific centers of the brain depends on how much sensory stimulation that center has received. The more developed a specific center in the brain is, the more pleasure can be obtained from employing the sensory activities related to that specific center because of the greater neurochemical producing capabilities of that center.

What does all this have to do with eating, becoming healthy and fit, and losing weight? As you might recall in Chapter 2, there is a center for eating in the hypothalamus. The more it is used and excited the larger it can become, and in someone with a large eating center, it can cause that person to enjoy eating more than doing other things. So every time we feel the need to elevate our mood we turn to what we know will help us feel better. If we train ourselves to receive pleasures from eating, then that is what we will do. If we can learn to receive pleasures from a variety of other activities besides eating, then it will become much easier to control the emotional factors associated with overeating. If we make it a habit to indulge ourselves in sports and recreational activities such as swimming, jogging, walking, dancing, singing, and anything else we might enjoy, then we will develop larger centers in the brain controlling these activities, and we will enjoy doing these activities as much as eating. The idea is to strike a balance of activities and release all the various neurochemicals that the body can produce to enhance our figures and modify our mood. When we have a varied source of endorphins in our bodies we feel happier, and the direct result of muscular activities will result in increasing body metabolism, giving us more energy and we will be able to burn all the fat the body can burn.

The amount of pleasure derived from an activity reinforces that activity. By choosing an activity that we enjoy, we will pursue that activity and incorporate it into our daily lifestyles, which will make our lives healthier and much more enjoyable.

Also, remember that we have satiation centers in the brain that bring about sensations of satiety after we have consumed the nutrients that are required in the body at the cellular level. When we eat for emotional gratification, we tend to ignore our satiation signals and continue eating. When we do not use our abilities we lose them. Therefore, it is quite conceivable to think that people who eat for emotional gratification will eventually develop a larger center of eating and a less developed center of satiation, and tend to eat without knowing when to stop. It is important that we become aware of when we are eating for emotional reasons, and practice responding to satiation signals.

Emotions and Food

When our bodies are well nourished we will be stronger physically and emotionally, and when we are stronger physically and emotionally we will be able to nourish ourselves more effectively. Our physical, emotional, and nutritional needs are closely related and interdependent. The "fight or flight" mechanisms require a tremendous boost of energy which becomes instantly available in the body to allow us to undertake tasks which normally would not be possible with existing levels of blood sugar. Such mechanisms utilize tremendous amounts of nutrients that must be replaced. Each emotion causes a different physiological effect within our bodies, calling for a wide spectrum of nutrients. How we cope with our emotional needs depends, at least in part, on how well nourished we are and how we go about obtaining the required nutrients. For example, when we encounter an emotional upheaval, our reaction depends on the momentary nutritional state of our body. If our body has enough stored energy when the need arises, we would probably react in a much more effective manner to solve the problem than if we were hungry.

Our emotional needs stem from our sensory feelings and are greatly associated with the amounts of endorphins we are capable of manufacturing. Metabolic imbalances are often the result of the body attempting to adapt to the crises it encounters. To avert emotional crises and maintain physical well-being, we should strengthen our emotional state by increasing our physical and social activities and by becoming more responsive to our physical and dietary needs. People who do not get enough satisfaction and joy from their work or relationships tend to ignore their physical and emotional feelings, finding consolation and pleasure in food and eating instead (Selye, 1956). It becomes futile to attempt to lose weight without focusing on the physical, emotional, and nutritional components of our health and treating ourselves as a whole, entitled to being satisfied and content in all aspects of our lives.

Chapter 6

Sensory Eating Mechanisms

Sensory Organs and The Mechanisms That Control Eating

All sensory organs have an important role to play in maintaining our nutritional health and well-being. With our eyes we examine the food we eat. The sight of food has a great impact on triggering hunger sensations. The sense of touch detects the texture and palatability of the food. The sense of hearing plays an important role also. We recognize the sounds of various foods such as the crunch of an apple or the sizzling sound of frying. Any of these stimuli can whet our appetites. However, the senses of taste and smell have the most important role in the mechanisms which control eating. The taste and the smell of food stimulate the flow of digestive juices and induce pleasurable or objectionable sensations according to the food we eat.

Recent studies on the senses of taste and smell reveal that many eating behaviors are associated with the sense of taste and the sense of smell. It has been found that humans can distinguish tens of thousands of different odours directly associated with eating, and distinguish the taste of all the foods that we eat.

The strategic location of the organs of taste and smell

are most revealing to the importance of their functions. They are situated at the gates of food and air intake. Food and odors must come in contact with these two organs before entering the body. When any food or smell is not acceptable, the gagging reflexes and nausea are triggered so the undesirable foods are rejected.

Ten thousand taste buds, each one having fifty receptor cells, are strategically positioned at the gate of the digestive system. They are spread out on the surface of the tongue, the roof of the mouth and the throat. Their primary objective is to monitor all substances that enter our bodies. Taste buds are very discriminatory and change their preferences in relation to the body's needs. Before any food substance can be tasted, it must dissolve in the saliva of the mouth, and diffuse into the taste bud. Highly diffusible substances such as salt and other small compounds are recognized more readily than the larger molecules like proteins and fat. Until recently, it was believed that different taste buds existed for each taste of salt, sweet, sour, and bitter. Science magazine reports that:

> Researchers working with mud puppies - a variety of salamanders with large taste buds - made detailed recordings from individual taste buds. Their studies indicated that taste buds are not merely passive recordings of chemical reactions in the mouth. The taste neurons communicate with each other in complex ways, even within a single taste bud, before sending their sensory message to the brain. "Like flavor sensitive microprocessors, specialized nerve clusters 'make decisions' about what they are experiencing" says Steven D. Roper of Colorado State University in Fort Collins.
>
> The classical view that taste buds come in only four

basic varieties appears oversimplified. New evidence indicates that each individual taste bud contains about 40 taste sensitive cells and can detect and recognize the various combinations of all the components of the foods we eat (Weiss, 1989).

Taste buds communicate and transmit messages back and forth between themselves, and then communicate their findings to the center of taste in the hypothalamus. Nerve pathways also connect the taste buds to the higher centers of the cortex.

If taste buds can communicate amongst themselves perhaps they are analysing the food they are tasting.

Eh hum yes...that is a fat molecule....What have you got there Charlie? Oh Buddy I think I hit a glucose molecule! Sweety here beside me is certain he has detected a carbohydrate molecule. Listen Buddy; between you and me I suspect our owner is eating a doughnut! We better call Madam Neuron upstairs and give her the news...

Of course this is a far-fetched conversation. What could ten thousand taste buds communicate amongst themselves? What could the more than 40 microprocessing cells in each taste bud distinguish? Imagine a border patrol inspecting each and every molecule of food we eat, identifying every pulverized and ground morsel of food that enters our mouths, and transferring the gathered information into memory banks in the brain. Otherwise, why would there be such elaborate nerve pathways transmitting taste impulses within the nervous system (see fig. 6).

The senses of taste and smell play a much greater

role than just simply analyzing food to determine if it is sweet, sour, bitter, salty, enjoyable or disgusting. These organs have a key role in accepting or rejecting the foods that enter the body. They also play a role in helping to keep an inventory of the foods consumed, helping us to choose the foods we eat. Why is it that a person craving for certain food can almost taste and smell that food? Why do taste buds keep changing their preferences for foods according to the momentary needs of our bodies?

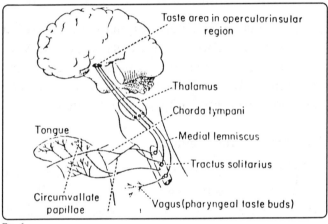

Fig. 6
Nerve pathways between the tastebuds and the brain

A sweet taste is usually pleasant, causing an animal to choose foods that are sweet. It indicates that fruit is ripe or nutritious. A bitter taste is generally unpleasant. Sour and salty tastes are sometimes pleasant and sometimes unpleasant. The pleasantness of tastes is indicated by how much of a certain food is consumed. Once we eat all that we want of a certain food we stop liking that food for a while, and when we have not eaten a certain type of food for a while we start to crave it. Our like and dislike of food is determined by the momentary nutritional state of the body. Foods needed by the body at the cellular level tend to taste more delicious. Our preferences for the taste of food changes according to the demands of our bodies. Certain foods taste more pleasant when our cells are demanding specific nutrients, allowing us to vary our diet according to the momentary needs of our bodies.

What Causes Sensations of Hunger and Satiation?

There are several proposals put forward as to what causes a person to feel hungry or satiated. Most of these proposals are based on signals arriving to the brain from various locations in the gastrointestinal tract, and other organs instigating hunger or satiation.

Distention of the Stomach

The fullness or emptiness of the stomach is one of the triggers of satiety or hunger. The discomfort of a distended stomach after eating a big meal will cause a person to stop eating temporarily. A growling stomach reminds a person that gases are moving in the intestines and perhaps it is time to eat. From personal experience, we know that eating a calorie-rich meal is more fulfilling than a calorie-reduced meal. You may recall Dr. Fomon's experiment in Chapter 1 in which babies receiving calorie-reduced meals increased their food intake in direct proportion to the calorie reduction. Perhaps the distention of the stomach does not have much to do with feeling satiated, but discomfort might prevent us from eating more.

Perhaps a distended stomach causes satiation indirectly, for a distended stomach triggers the secretion of digestive juices in the small intestine. Many theories suggest that satiation can be caused by the amounts of digestive juices secreted.

Blood Sugar Levels

When glucose levels in the blood are reduced, a person feels hungry. When glucose levels rise, satiety is maintained. However, there is a slight flaw in this theory. Hunger is triggered by specific receptors in the brain that detect a fall in blood sugar levels, while satiety occurs when the food is still in the stomach and has not reached the blood yet. Therefore, the feeling of satiation during a meal could not have been triggered by a rise in blood sugar levels. There must be some other reason why we feel satiated while the food is still in the stomach.

The Rate of Energy Production in the Cells

Our cells produce energy by burning carbon molecules. When our bodies are short of nutrients, the rate of conversion is affected. This, in turn, is transferred to the hunger and satiety centers in the brain, causing sensations of hunger when the rate of conversion is slower and satiety when the rate of conversion speeds up. This theory also has its flaws. Satiation occurs while the food is still in the stomach and has not yet reached the cells.

The Taste Bud Theory

Taste buds identify the foods we eat and through the process of transferring the information to the brain, various neurochemicals are released. The release of these neurochemicals is instantaneous and can influence the feelings of satiation when the food is still in the digestive tract. Perhaps a combination of all these factors has a role in initiating satiety.

How the Body Seeks Required Nutrients

Our bodies are designed to regulate and seek the nutrients they require. The hypothalamus receives input from many sensory organs such as taste, smell, as well as other internal senses that monitor our blood sugar and all other mineral and nutritive requirements at the cellular level. The job of the hypothalamus is to regulate and maintain homeostatic condition, by ensuring the availability of all required nutrients in the fluids surrounding the cells of the body.

Claude Bernard, a nineteenth century biologist, recognized the presence of extracellular fluid in and around the cells and referred to it as *Milieu Interne*, the internal environment. Sir Walter Canon, thirty years later, referred to the maintenance of the constant conditions of these fluids as homeostasis. Almost every organ in our bodies controls one or more of these fluid constituents. For instance, the circulatory system composed of the heart and the blood vessels transport blood and dissolved nutrients to all parts of the body reaching every cell. It is estimated that no cell is further away than 0.01 cm from a capillary of a blood vessel. Nutrients diffuse back and forth between the blood and the extracellular fluids, removing waste and bringing nourishment that the cells require to function. No fluid in the body remains unmixed for more than a few minutes. When a cell needs a certain element or nutrient, the cell can readily find the needed element or nutrient in the extracellular fluids in which it is bathed.

For example, suppose that a man accidentally cut his finger and it bled a considerable amount. His blood would form a clot and plug the cut. Free calcium in the extracellular fluid was used to form the clot. In turn, the calcium in the extracellular fluid would be replaced by the blood.

Calcium levels must remain at a constant level in the blood. Even the slightest drop in calcium levels would have severe consequences, including muscle cramps. Severe cramps in the diaphragm, the major breathing muscle, can hamper breathing, and depending on the severity of calcium shortage, can cause suffocation.

The parathyroid hormone is responsible for maintaining the blood calcium levels at a constant level. A slight drop in blood calcium levels causes the release of this hormone. The parathyroid glands are four little clusters found at the four corners of the thyroid gland situated in the throat (beside the Adam's apple). Within seconds of its release parathyroid hormone starts to work, conserving the body's supply of calcium. It prevents the kidneys from excreting any calcium in the urine, and activates large bones to release calcium from their structures. Calcium levels return to normal almost instantly and danger is averted.

Meanwhile, there is a center in the hypothalamus monitoring the whole episode. Perhaps it works by recording the amount of parathyroid hormone or the calcium levels in the blood. The task of these hypothalamic cells is to maintain the internal environment. This vital part of the brain is connected to various centers, allowing it to regulate all the internal functions of temperature control, food and fluid intake, water balance, and it also influences the endocrine system. It records what is needed, maintaining inventories of nutrients required by the body. Then it relates the requisitions to the higher regions of the brain to formalize them as a thought and craving. In the case of the bleeding man, his hypothalamic center keeps tabs on everything that is happening in his body, and cross-references this information with memory banks regarding what changes must come about to regulate homeostasis. What foods he should eat and when? How much? Perhaps the bleeding man will crave a glass of milk if he practices replacing calcium in his body with milk. He might crave for cabbage if he has learned to obtain his calcium by eating cabbage. The calcium lost during bleeding must be replaced. How will he know how much milk to drink or how much cabbage to eat? The hypothalamus in his brain has the records of how much calcium he has lost and his taste buds monitor the calcium he receives and convey their findings to the hypothalamus. As soon as the requisition for calcium is filled the appetite for milk or cabbage is relieved.

Chapter 7

How The Body Utilizes Energy

Energy Use in The Body

All body cells must have a constant and uninterrupted energy supply at all times. Without energy our cells die. Our bodies have two kinds of energy storage systems. One is glucose based, in which all carbohydrates and sugars absorbed from our diet are converted to glycogen, stored in the liver, and are then burned in the body as glucose. Glucose is the only source of fuel for brain cells. The other system is fat based. Fat is the main source of energy normally used by our muscles. Fat is absorbed from the gastrointestinal tract and is stored in the body as fat. Body fat breaks down to yield 90% fatty acids and 10% glycerol. This 10 % glycerol can be converted to glucose in the liver and sustain the brain cells in a small way during famine. During short periods of fasting our bodies spare their glucose and rely on fat for energy. During long fasts, our bodies rely upon other mechanisms to ensure the energy requirements for the brain. Eventually, during extended fasts, our bodies produce new glucose by dismantling body tissues and organs. When we are feasting, however, our bodies spare fat and obtain their energy from glucose.

We store larger amounts of fat. Our bodies house enough fat for up to two months or more to supply the energy needs of muscles. We store much smaller quantities of glucose, in the form of glycogen in the liver. We only store enough sugar for four hours of energy supply for the brain.

All our body cells except our brain cells are able to burn fatty acids and glucose interchangeably. Brain cells rely on blood glucose as their sole source of energy. Our brain cells receive their nutrition in a different way than the rest of our cells. Glial cells in the brain tissue are responsible for processing energy for the nerve cells. Glial cell membranes are mainly constructed of water based proteins and contain almost no fat and they are very delicate. Glial cells are not able to accommodate large molecules of fatty acids. These cells can allow only the smaller, water soluble glucose molecules to enter through their delicate membranes. Conversely, muscle cells cannot use glucose for energy without the aid of the hormone insulin because muscle cell membranes are composed of fat molecules and will repel water based glucose molecules.

Insulin is released from the Islet of Langerhans in the Pancreas and its job is to disperse and lower the blood sugar levels by forcing muscles to burn glucose instead of fat. Insulin also prevents fatty acids from leaving fat cells so that our bodies first utilize all the sugar that we have consumed in our meal.

We are able to store about three to four hundred calories of glycogen in the liver that will be converted into blood glucose as needed. This is a sufficient supply of energy for our brain to last us during our eight hours of sleep, and four hours when awake.

Although we have a two-month supply of spare energy in the form of fat, we cannot survive on burning fat alone. It is essential that people eat regularly about every three to four hours to ensure an uninterrupted supply of glucose energy to the brain.

We are also unable to store minerals, vitamins, and proteins on a long term basis. Therefore, eating regularly ensures the constant replenishment of these nutrients as well.

Although glucose is an important energy source and we cannot survive without respectable blood sugar levels, levels that are higher than 120 mg per 100 ml of glucose in the blood can cause many complications.

Diabetics suffer from the inability to regulate their blood sugar and their insulin production is affected. Their blood sugar levels rise above the desired 120 mg per 100 ml and can fall below 70 mg per 100 ml. High levels of blood sugar combined with acetone and other residue from the breaking down of body proteins irritate the very delicate vascular systems in the body. Damage may occur to the retina of the eye causing blindness, or to the fine lining of kidney tubules leading to kidney failure. Damage to the many fine blood vessels in the brain and the coronary artery may lead to stroke and myocardial infarction (heart attack) caused by a lack of blood supply to the heart muscle.

The hormone insulin plays a key role in maintaining a safe blood sugar level so that high amounts of blood sugar cannot cause any harm. After a meal, when the blood sugar level starts to rise, insulin is released. *Insulin acts on our body cells and stops the cells from using fat for energy until all the sugars ingested in a meal are metabolized.* (Either burned as fuel or stored as glycogen.)

When the blood sugar level begins to fall below 70 mg per 100 ml another hormone is released. This hormone, called *glucagon* has exactly the opposite effect of insulin. It stimulates the glycogen from the liver to be converted back to glucose and raise the blood glucose level. Glucagon also stimulates fat cells to release fatty acids and allows the body to resume burning fatty acids for our energy needs. When we constantly nibble on candies and sweets we will constantly maintain a steady stream of insulin in our system which will prevent fatty acids from ever leaving our fat cells. This causes our bodies to receive our energy mostly from burning glucose, preventing the burning of our body fat.

What Stops The Body From Burning Fat?

The hormone insulin stops the body from burning fat. *The primary stimulus for increased insulin secretion is the increase of blood glucose concentration, and the taste of sweet.* The release of insulin is a negative feedback mechanism between the pancreatic cells and the concentration of glucose in the blood flowing in them. The more glucose in the blood, the more insulin is produced. As soon as we eat, our body reacts and produces insulin to deal with the sugars found in a meal.

Also the amount of insulin released in our bodies is regulated according to the sweet taste we experience when we eat. In the experiment conducted by LeBlanc and Cabanac (Chapter 1), it was found that eating a sugar pie, chewing it, then spitting it out without swallowing raised the metabolic rate. This experiment indicates that *our bodies respond to eating as soon as we taste food,* almost instantly, while it is still in our mouth. We know from our own experiences that our mouth waters at the sight, smell, sound, and thought of food or when we are about to eat something nice. Our reaction to food causes the release of digestive juices. All of this indicates that our mechanisms which control eating are triggered by sensory messages and even the movements involved during eating. The rise in metabolic rate is triggered not by the food alone, but also by the increased activities of our bodies, such as preparing digestive juices and hormones in response to the anticipation of eating.

Other experiments indicate that *the mere taste of the foods eaten, regardless of the caloric value of the food itself, causes the release of insulin.* Tordoff (1988) found that rats given saccharin (an artificial, non-caloric sweetener) to drink before their meal increased their food intake by 10 to 15 percent. Brala and Hagen (1983) conducted an experiment in which university students were given milkshakes, some sweetened with sugar and others sweetened with artificial sweetener. One half of the students were asked to rinse their mouth with a solution of gymnemic acid, a chemical that blocks sweet taste, prior to drinking the milkshakes. Some students consumed sugar and some consumed artificial sweetener with their milkshakes, and fifty percent of the students drank their milkshakes without being able to taste sweet. Ninety minutes later, all the students were offered snacks. Students who had tasted a sweet milkshake reported being hungrier than those who could not taste sweet due to the gymnemic acid. The students who tasted artificial sweetener in their milkshake were equally hungry as students who had sugar sweetened milkshakes. *A logical deduction is that students who experienced the sweet taste felt hungrier because their blood sugar levels dropped more than the students who could not taste the sweet in the milkshake. This is most likely due to the taste of sweet they have experienced which caused the release of insulin. The Students who could not taste sweet would have not released insulin because there was no sensory experience of sweetness to trigger the release of insulin.*

An explanation for the sweet tasters' lowered blood sugar was that the taste of sweet triggered the release of insulin, and shifted their metabolism to burn glucose instead of fat, thus lowering blood sugar levels, and consequently making them feel hungry shortly after eating. This is similar to the rats mentioned above, who experienced the taste of saccharin before their meal, ate 15% more and gained weight. It is most likely that the taste of sweet triggered the release of insulin and caused a lowering of blood sugar levels which subsequently triggered hunger sensations causing the rats to eat more.

Our bodies react to the artificial sweetness and sugar sweetness in the same manner, even though artificial sweeteners do not raise our blood sugar levels. Taste buds have the ability to identify the molecular structure of the foods we eat. Food chemists have studied sugar and other sweet tasting substances and identified the exact arrangement of the atoms in these molecules that stimulate the sweet taste receptors on the surface of the tongue. Their findings indicate that all sweet tasting molecular structures, including artificial sweeteners have the same features. It is difficult for a taste bud to differentiate between artificial, calorie-free sweetness and sucrose sweetness.

The artificial sweetener industry has succeeded in producing a sweet taste that is identical to sucrose but without the calories. These artificial sweeteners fool our taste buds and we react to the taste of these sweeteners in the same way we react to the taste of sugar, by releasing insulin.

These diet sweeteners are fine for diabetics because their tasting of sweet will not trigger the release of insulin in the same way as it would for non-diabetics. But when non-diabetic persons experience the taste of sweet from artificial sweeteners, they react as if they have tasted sugar, resulting in a shift in their metabolism to burn glucose instead of fat. Thus the blood sugar level is lowered and they end up feeling hungry shortly afterwards.

When we subject ourselves to the taste of sweet, sometimes with real sugar which will raise our blood sugar levels, and other times from artificial sweeteners, which do not raise blood sugar but their sweet taste triggers the release of insulin, and drastically reduces blood sugar levels, we will thoroughly confuse our insulin producing mechanisms.

In addition to blood glucose concentration there are other factors that regulate the release of insulin. For example, after a high protein meal, where there is an elevated level of amino acids in the blood, the level of insulin also increases. The release of insulin promotes protein synthesis by the cells and lowers blood amino acids.

Also the digestive system releases gastrointestinal hormones, in response to the presence of food in the digestive tract. These hormones have been shown to stimulate insulin release and are called Glucose-dependent Insulinotrophic Peptides (GIP). These peptides initiate the release of insulin in anticipation of a meal, *before nutrient absorption increases the concentration of glucose in the blood.*

Dieting and Exercise Are Counterproductive

Dieting and exercise are counterproductive and do not necessarily lead to weight loss. Manifestoes declaring that the secrets of losing weight are dieting and exercise are not quite accurate. When people first begin to exercise, their muscles are not well equipped to burn large amounts of fat, nor are their lungs and circulatory systems capable of delivering the oxygen required to burn fat in large quantities. When people first embark on an exercise program, their muscles will draw some of their energy for the exercise from blood glucose, not from fat. If one is restricting one's carbohydrate intake, in many instances the brain is left short of energy. The body resorts to breaking down fatty acids to acetone to provide energy for brain cells. Not all brain cells are able to use acetone, and we start to breakdown body cells to convert the carbon molecules in these cells to glucose to supply the brain cells with glucose. Therefore, restricting calorie intake and exercising at the same time becomes counterproductive and self-defeating. Besides lowering body metabolism, the ordeal of offering the brain cells acetone results in a negative conditioning, causing a psychological dislike of exercise. The secret to enjoying exercising is to exercise without dieting and strive to develop our muscles to draw their energy totally from burning fat.

Our bodies learn to adjust fuel consumption according to the patterns of our regular daily routines. An average healthy body stores some glycogen in the liver for the exclusive use of brain cells and stores some glycogen in the muscles to be used for quick energy needs. Of course there are large quantities of fuel supplies in the form of fat that can be released during exercise. Muscles can burn large quantities of fat during exercise, but there is a trick to it. For the muscles to burn large quantities of fat there must be enough supplies of oxygen to break down the large carbon chains of fat molecules. Also, there must be enough mitochondria developed in the muscle cells to effectively facilitate the burning of fat. Mitochondria are organelles (literally "little organs") within a cell where metabolic reactions occur. They are the fireplaces in the cells where combustion takes place.

When we first begin to exercise, fatty acids are released from our fat cells and enter our muscles where they are broken down to release energy. Fatty acids need a steady supply of oxygen to continue the process of combustion. Our lungs and cardiovascular system must first develop so they can keep delivering a steady supply of oxygen to keep fat burning in the mitochondria of our muscle cells. Glucose, on the other hand, can be burned anaerobically (without oxygen), forming lactic acid. During intense exercise, when muscle cells require massive energy quickly, muscles start to burn glucose from the glycogen stored in the muscles and then begin to draw glucose from the blood to continue the release of energy.

Lactic acid build-up in the muscles causes stiffness which develops into pain until the lactic acid is dissipated after a few days. We have often experienced such pain when we first start on an exercise program, join an aerobics class, or start playing tennis. The first few sessions of exercise cause a general muscle stiffness and pain until the muscles develop more mitochondria, allowing muscles to burn fat more easily.

When the muscles develop more mitochondria, when the lungs improve their capacity to better oxygenate the blood, and the cardiovascular system becomes capable of delivering enough oxygen to the cells, then muscles will burn fat freely, and we will be able to exercise for longer periods of time without developing muscle pain. When muscles are receiving their energy from burning fat, we will feel energetic, and we will not feel hungry, because our blood sugar levels will not become depleted. We will be left with a good supply of blood sugar reserved exclusively for the brain.

Novices might plunge into an exercise and weight loss program with great enthusiasm, determined to lose every inch of body fat, then find themselves fatigued quickly. They would almost certainly develop muscle aches and pains if not prepared. This, combined with low carbohydrate intake, will cause development of ketosis (breaking of fatty acids into ketone bodies or acetone) which leads to a lowered metabolism. Instead of losing weight, they will end up with a lowered metabolism, and will likely gain more weight. These people will end up tormenting themselves without any benefit whatsoever. When their muscles use up their brain fuel and leave their brain cells without nutrients, they will become irritable. This, combined with the aches and pains they suffer from lactic acid-build up, will lead them to avoid exercising. This is known as *negative conditioning* to exercise.

It is important that we start with warm-up exercises, because warm-up exercises give our bodies time to mobilize fatty acids in preparation for more vigorous exercises to follow. During warm-up exercises our muscles can burn fat slowly and spare muscle glycogen, reducing the extent of lactic acid build-up in the muscle which results in stiffness, muscle pain, and injury.

When we begin an exercise program, for the first week or so, our appetite will increase and we will feel hungry after exercising. This is because muscles use the energy from blood glucose, lowering the blood sugar levels, and causing the release of neurochemicals that trigger our sensations of hunger.

When our muscles become efficient fat burners and draw their energy from burning fat, then hunger sensations after exercise subside, because our muscles derive their energy from fat, which is abundantly available (even in slim people!), without depleting the blood sugar that is reserved for the brain.

When we begin to exercise, the release of insulin is suppressed in our bodies because of the release of stress hormones, epinephrine, cortisol, and thyroid. These stress hormones allow for an increase in both blood glucose, and fatty acid levels without an increase in insulin. This allows our muscles to continue to burn fat.

When our bodies are able to meet the energy requirements of our cells, we will not release any insulin. We can go for long hours exercising without feeling fatigued, and our blood glucose levels will not become depleted. Our brain will continue receiving its ample share of glucose from the blood and manufacture the endorphins that make us feel good. Prolonged exercise will also allow the release of endorphins giving us a Runners' High.

We do not have to run to get a dose of the good feeling experienced from the release of endorphins. Walking, swimming, skipping, playing tennis, and any other exercise carried out over thirty minutes, which uses the large muscles of the buttocks, abdomen, and thighs, will result in an increased endorphin release. Our metabolism will rise, allowing us to feel even more energetic after many hours of exercise. After exercise we experience an invigorating sensation that makes us feel glad we are alive. This good feeling compels us to like exercise and to continue exercising on a regular basis.

The Illusion of Quick Weight Loss Diets

When the glycogen reserves in the liver become depleted and we continue a restricted carbohydrate diet in order to lose weight, our bodies start to seek alternate means to sustain our brain cells. Our bodies resort to internal "self-cannibalism". We start to break down our own body cells to provide energy for the brain. At this point, the cannibalism really kicks in. Our bodies begin to break down the cells of muscles, liver, and spleen to extract their protein. Excess nitrogen from this breakdown is expelled in the urine, while the remainder of the broken down cells are converted to glucose in order to feed the brain cells. This breakdown process is called ketosis. The debris from the broken down tissues is uric acid which accumulates in the blood, and together with ketone bodies is processed by the kidneys and extracted into the urine. That is why the urine of a starved person smells strong. Acetone also evaporates from the lungs, giving the breath of a starved person a sour smell tinged with a mildew-like odour. This foul smelling breath is a sure sign that we have approached a stage where our metabolism is slowing and our brain is sustained by acetone. The brain is short of energy and will not be able to produce the neurochemicals that activate our metabolic activities, and most of these activities slow down to minimum levels.

All fad diets that lead to ketosis predispose a person to become susceptible to weight gain. Many people who follow these diets are deceived and taken aback by the illusion of the large amounts of weight loss registered on the scale during the first few days of their regime. The scales do not differentiate between loss of fat, water or protein. During starvation and crash diets, when the brain is sustained by acetone, we may experience weight loss. But, it is mostly water, minerals, and protein that are lost from our organs - not fat! As soon as we start to eat as we ate prior to dieting, our bodies quickly return to their original weight. A raging hunger sets in to compel us to replace the required nutrients, and we start to eat without discrimination. All water and minerals lost during our dieting are quickly replaced and we gain back weight as quickly as we had lost it.

People who feed their brain acetone will eventually discover that it will become progressively harder for them to lose weight and easier to gain it. Besides metabolic and weight-related consequences, feeding the brain acetone has more far-reaching detrimental effects on mood, behavior, and alertness. Studies indicate that the frequency of automobile accidents and many other industrial accidents which require alertness are greater during long-term calorie reduced diets. If we do not drink enough water, the kidneys can become blocked and permanently damaged due to the metabolic debris accumulated in the blood during starvation. Drinking large quantities of water is a must during calorie-reduced diets, and it will prevent kidney damage if we drink these recommended quantities. However, feeding the brain acetone is what causes our body to lower its metabolic reactions, rendering us susceptible to weight gain.

Be Aware Of Fruity Smelling Breath

Dieters today say that when their breath begins to smell fruity sweet, it is an encouraging sign. It means that their body is burning fat. Yes, when our breath begins to smell fruity, our bodies are burning fat and breaking down fatty acids to acetone to feed our brain. Our bodies are also sacrificing our muscle, spleen, and liver tissue by drawing the proteins out of their cells, to convert them to glucose, for feeding the brain which cannot survive on acetone.

What is so encouraging about burning up our own organs and muscle cells? Muscle cells are the major fat burners in our bodies. If muscles are burned and wasted, how are we going to burn fat? Our body organs are the main centers for metabolic functions and heat production. Once our organs lose their tissue, how will we maintain our body temperature? How will we continue metabolic functions? When we lose important tissues and muscles, our metabolism is lowered.

When our bodies shift to burning acetone for brain fuel a dangerous and very deceiving phenomenon occurs. When ketone bodies appear, our hunger disappears, our thinking becomes clearer. We experience a calm, more focused state of mind. These signs encourage us to continue starving ourselves. Combined with the dramatic readings of weight loss as told by the scale during the first week of dieting, we become encouraged that our diet is working and continue the foolishness.

The reason an energy deprived person's hunger disappears is because their body has slowed down its metabolic activities. Our bodies know that to search for food requires more energy, and energy is scarce. The reason our mind becomes clearer and more focused is probably because most of our metabolic functions have slowed down, so we feel cold and sleepy, refrain from thinking, and fewer sensory messages will be triggered by internal functions. Essentially, our bodies are in a crisis. Most autonomic brain activities relating to metabolism are geared down, leaving more scope for cognitive thoughts. This is what monks experience when they fast.

When we are dieting and restricting our food intake, we start to lose body fluids, body tissue, important minerals and water, and we will record up to a ten pound loss in our body weight within a short period of time ranging from several days to a few weeks. We will feel good about what we are doing. Our disappointment comes later, when we start to eat. All of a sudden we will gain weight in direct proportions to the losses we have maintained at the start of our diet, and perhaps a little more. By no means does allowing our brain to survive on scraps of fatty acids reduce our weight on a permanent basis. If we fast for a few days, then return to eating, we will develop a raging appetite until our nutritive stores are replenished and we will end up gaining more weight than before we started our diet. Repeated attempts at yo-yo dieting can mercilessly render us prone to weight gain.

A Lean, Mean, Fat Burning Machine

In order for our muscles to burn large quantities of fat, all body mechanisms must work hand in hand to ensure the proper conditions conducive to burning fat. By no means we will be able to burn our body fat when we do not have the proper energy to supply our brain cells, so that they can produce the neurochemicals necessary to carry out the business of living. Remember it is the neurochemicals released in our bodies that control every action and reaction of the body. Our bodies are designed to function automatically, in cause and effect sequences, through the actions of these neurochemicals and hormones. When any one system is not working at its full capacity, it will affect all the other systems of the body.

Our muscles are capable of burning unlimited quantities of fat provided that all other systems and organs in our bodies are doing their jobs. It is important that the heart and the circulatory system are well developed to supply the nutrients and oxygen to the muscles. Muscle cells, in turn, will increase the number of mitochondria in to provide the fireplaces where the burning will take place. Most importantly, our nervous system needs to receive the required nutrients to ensure the production of all the neurochemicals needed in order for the body metabolism to rise, initiating demands to burn body fat.

When we develop our lungs to supply the oxygen required, and our cardiovascular system to pump the nutrients and the oxygen to the muscles, and when our brain cells have the share of energy they need, then there will be no need for the release of insulin in the body, and our muscles will burn every molecule of fat that becomes available to them.

We all know that fire needs oxygen to burn and burning our body fat is no exception. Fire will not start if there is not enough ventilation. Our body's ventilation system consists of our lungs and our cardiovascular system, which ensures the supply of oxygen to our body cells.

Muscles were made to burn fat. Physical exercise is the only method that will develop the three components necessary to make our bodies efficient fat burners. These components are:

1- A super-efficient cardiovascular system to pump air and nutrients to the muscles.

2- Increased number of mitochondria within the muscles to facilitate the efficient burning that must take place to meet the required energy needs.

3- Adequate nutrients must be constantly available to all body cells including brain cells, so that our body cells can build and repair themselves and carry on their work, thus ensuring healthy cells capable of functioning adequately.

To develop our bodies into efficient fat burners, it is essential that we exercise on a regular basis, and find enjoyment while exercising. Exercise must be taken seriously and prepared for, otherwise we can injure ourselves and find pain that will easily deter us from exercising. We should wear proper shoes, comfortable loose clothing, and most importantly, choose an exercise that we enjoy. Start to exercise at a very slow pace, increasing intensity gradually. It is necessary to give ourselves enough time to strengthen our muscles and slowly improve our cardiovascular capacity. The key to maintaining exercise on a regular basis is to refrain from restricting calories until our muscles develop their ability to burn fat freely. This will ensure that our brain is not left short of nutrients. We will know that we are receiving our energy from burning fat when we are able to exercise for much longer periods of time and more intensively, without feeling hungry or exhausted. We will feel energetic after exercise because our blood sugar remains within the normal range during exercise. Our metabolism will rise and we will produce neurochemicals that will make us feel good about ourselves and enjoy exercising. The glucose supplies in our bodies will be reserved for our brain cells only. Meanwhile, muscle cells will draw 100% of their energy requirements from fat.

Yo-yo style exercising on and off for a few days, every now and then, has little effect on developing mitochondria in the muscles. Once we stop exercising, our muscles start to shrink. Our bodies have a rule: Use it or lose it. Any muscle, tissue, organ, or mechanism of the body that is not used deteriorates and is lost. If we do not use our muscles for a few weeks, our muscles begin to waste away.

Regular exercise trains the muscles to become efficient fat burners. Once we develop our muscles to burn fat effectively then there will be no stopping. Muscles will start to burn every molecule of fat that comes near them. Our metabolic rate will rise, and sooner than we know it, body fat will disappear, turning our bodies into lean, mean, fat burning machines. The tables will turn! Instead of pondering if we should eat a speck of food or not, we will eat whatever we want to eat, and without guilt or fear of not being able to balance our energy intake to our energy output. We will be able to eat whatever we *feel* we want to eat and our bodies will utilize it and still maintain our energy balance without gaining weight.

In Chapter 1, we mentioned that there are some

people who seem to have bodies that are able to adjust weight with little conscious effort. Well, people who can eat whatever they want and not gain weight are people who have muscles that can draw their energy 100 per cent from burning fat, leaving the blood sugar energy exclusively for their brain. They eat what they want and when they want; and whatever they eat their muscles are capable of burning.

In the beginning, when we start to exercise, it is a good idea to refrain from weighing ourselves. When we start to develop muscles, we might even gain some weight, as muscles are heavier than fat. In most instances the muscles are developing and the fat layers are disappearing. It is very disappointing and counterproductive to trust the scales to measure our progress. If we still feel compelled to measure our progress by measuring our bodies, despite the fact that exercise makes us *feel* great, we should try on clothing that used to be snug before starting the exercise program. The goal is to feel good and look good, to become healthy and fit, not emaciated and sickly. As long as we are reaching our goal of looking and feeling good, we need not worry about weight loss. Our bodies will maintain the desirable weight on their own terms.

Chapter 8

Pleasure Seeking

The Magic Ride in Search of Pleasure

The magic ride through evolutionary history was constantly empowered by the desire to experience pleasure, the ability to feel pleasure, and the capacity to learn and adapt to maintain the feelings of pleasure. The ability to retract from pain allowed organisms to exist, but the desire to seek pleasure has guided the living organism to treasure life and adapt to find enjoyment in living. We sometimes think that life is not worth living when we are not enjoying ourselves.

The ability to feel is the most important tool that living organisms have. It is the ability to feel that allows the organism to maintain and value its life. All living organisms are equipped with sensory mechanisms which detect all aspects of their environment. These mechanisms are designed to defend the living organism and ensure its survival. The mechanisms of survival have developed from a simple system of learning to avoid pain and seek the conditions that bring about pleasure. Even the simplest form of life, bacteria, has learned to form spores and protect itself from an adverse environment, emerging later by letting down its guard in favorable conditions. In more advanced life forms, protective mechanisms developed based on the sensory perception of pain and pleasure.

In the evolutionary development of man, simple defensive mechanisms that were apparent in lower life forms became controlled by a much more complex nervous system. This system progressed from a simple nerve fiber connecting different parts of the body found in primitive multicellular animals, to a very complex nervous system containing twelve billion neurons in human beings.

During the first stages of the evolution of the nervous system, a neuronal axis was formed along the body of lower organisms, which later developed into the spinal cord. Then there developed in the head end of the neuronal axis an enlarged collection of neurons which transmitted control signals down to all parts of the body. This is the type of nervous system we find in fish, reptiles, and birds. The reptilian and avian nervous system can be compared to the basal regions of the human brain. A final stage of evolutionary development of the brain was an overgrowth of the nervous tissue surrounding the brain's basal regions, as seen primarily in mammals, reaching a very advanced level in humans.

While new functions were evolving, older functions remained common between the lowest animal and man. For example, the reflex response in an earthworm is represented as the reflex action in man. However, in man it is controlled almost entirely by the spinal cord. The ability to navigate in birds and fish is through the development of the equilibrium process which is also present in man. Our equilibrium mechanism is controlled by the basal regions of the brain, while the same mechanism in the fish is in the highest region of the fish brain. Mammals developed certain mental abilities to store information as memory and use this memory throughout life. The human brain developed even further when it became associated with vast storage of memory and a more complex process of learning and thinking. Along with learning and thinking came the art of communicating. We learned to communicate through language, vision, sound, and touch which allowed humans to discover the joy of relating to one another, and sharing their experiences.

The Need To Experience Pleasure

Pleasure seeking is the most important tool the body has to help the individual to survive among the agony and the turmoil that living can offer. We like to receive joy and happiness in everything that we do; it is our reward for living. The environmental conditions that we live in can be harsh and unpleasant. The business of living does not come without pain. For example, the day to day activities cause body cells to endure friction. This is wear and tear that can eventually result in destruction of tissues. Wounds sustained by nicks and bruises often become infected. This can cause pain that will stop the individual from continuing important living tasks, such as seeking food, running away from danger, attacking in self-defense, mating or other things. Pain can definitely hinder and paralyse our ability and resolve.

An overwhelming sensation of separation and free fall is experienced when a baby first arrives into this hostile world, separated from the comforts of its mother's womb, facing a cold, harsh, unfamiliar world. This, coupled with a smack on its tiny little bottom, is enough to make it want to go right back to where it has come from. It is the pleasure experienced in sucking, feeding, and cuddling that encourages the little one to cope with adversities encountered early on in life. From then on, each and every step of the way, from the cradle to the grave, we battle with feelings of insecurity, fear, anger, physical and emotional pain, disappointments, and sadness. It is for this reason that we learn to seek the activities that will give us pleasure to overcome all adversities, and maintain cheerfulness and joy.

The human body is designed to receive joy by participating in activities that promote and enhance our lives. Imagine billions of neurons from all our sensory organs carrying a wealth of information to our brains from every corner of our bodies. Imagine what really happens in our bodies when we look out of the window and see the sun is shining, when we see the trees and the blue sky, when we hear the chirping of the birds, the rustling of the leaves, or the crashing of the waves on the shores, when we taste the sweet taste of honey or the wholesome taste of a nourishing soup that satisfies our hunger. We feel good. To feel good is a wonderful feeling we all like to experience. Sometimes we recall past events that gave us good feelings, and smile. The nerve pathways in our bodies are constantly transmitting messages and leaving behind "pleasure trails".

Pain, on the other hand is an unpleasant feeling which causes us to stop our action and withdraw from

Chapter 8

the painful source or activity. Pain sensations travel just like any other sensation. Pain also produces neuro-chemicals much the same way that any other message or sensation does. Pain-sensing neurons are found in almost all parts of our bodies. When these sensations travel to the brain, they reach a specific center for pain and the appropriate neurochemicals are released: specifically dopamine, which is a powerful pain relieving chemical and is as potent as morphine. Pain has an important role in delivering us from evil and harmful circumstances. Emotional, and other psychological perceptions of pain (documented by Sternbach, 1968) suggest the existence of neuronal mechanisms translating pain into unpleasant feelings. For example we all know first hand that we do not like to be punched. It hurts and makes us feel angry. We might retaliate and in future avoid the situation and the person who punched us. On the other hand we like the sensations of being massaged and touched gently. We enjoy the sensations and encourage the massage giver to continue the massage. We might even maneuver to stay close to this person in the hope of getting another massage.

The body has developed mechanisms to cope with pain. A considerable amount of neuronal circuitry is devoted to reduce pain to help us cope with the stress that life has to offer. Often the excitement and the surge of endorphins in the body can totally wipe out the pain temporarily. Beecher (1959) describes that American soldiers who fought in Anzio, Italy during World War II reported that they did not feel pain sustained during the battle. Similarly, football players often hurt themselves and continue the game without even realizing that they are injured. The body produces endogenous morphine like substances -endorphins and enkephalins- to block pain receptors from transmitting pain signals to the brain. It is not clear how the body's natural pain relieving chemicals are activated. Factors known to modulate the experience of pain include prolonged muscular exercise, and the awareness that painful circumstances are inescapable. For example, when an animal must endure pain to survive and the reduction of pain sensitivity is in the animal's best interest, the body releases endogenous morphines to soothe pain so that pain does not stand in the way of continuing important living tasks.

Pleasures In Sports and Recreational Activities

The combination of several sensory pathways activated simultaneously increases the stress placed on the body and triggers the release of endorphins, giving the person a natural high. To challenge all of his senses, a skier places himself in an inescapable position, testing his skill, his ability to maneuver down that slope without being hurt. Skiing challenges the sensations of equilibrium, sight, touch, hearing, and the coordination of these senses with speed and free fall. Skiers learn to control all the elements of danger associated with free fall. Experienced skiers are fully aware of their position on the hill in relation to their surroundings even at considerable speeds, maintaining full control, learning to execute each and every move with deliberation and precision. Tightening and loosening up leg muscles with each turn challenging all their muscles, joints, and senses, and gracefully swaying from side to side and descending down the slopes, skiers are totally absorbed in the art of skiing and having fun. Think how many endorphins are produced from the physical sensations that are traveling up and down the skiers' nerve pathways. This, combined with the endorphins produced by the mental picture of conquering the mountain, will give the skiers enough thrill to allow their pleasurable experiences to soar higher than the mountain down which they just skied.

Spectator sports give a different type of pleasure. For example, a soccer game or a football game gives the players and the spectators pleasure because in these games both players and spectators challenge themselves to win the game. Besides the physical aspects of the players pumping oxygen in to every cell of their body, endorphins are produced from stimuli reaching every muscle and joint. Team sports are built on an ultimate trust and confidence shared among the players, providing them with psychological pride and self-worth. It starts with each player focusing on his role in the play, then his attention moves to the other team-mates, forming a bond based on their trust in each other. The whole team becomes united as one. Each goal scored becomes glory for all. Even the spectators join in the process and identify themselves with their team, sharing a common trust and confidence. A united front of players and spectators play the game as one. Players probably receive the most pleasure, but spectators share the glory, perceiving themselves as playing too. Human beings enjoy relating to each other. They have a deep need to be able to communicate with each other, to reach each other, to trust and depend upon each other. They have a need to belong. Spectator sports provide all that. For the duration of the game, all those supporting fans consider themselves as one, they trust and agree with each other, even if it is just for the sake of the game. People from all walks of life, who would not even look at each other under different circumstances, cheer together and hug one another, especially if their team wins. Imagine how much fun they have.

Swimmers have fun in a different way. They challenge their senses of balance, coordination, and endurance, by placing themselves in a "sink or swim" position. Being submerged in water also has other soothing effects on mammals. It is reminiscent of the calm serenity experienced in the womb. The water gently surrounds the body and stimulates the billions of sensory receptors found on the surface of the skin. Swimming also requires muscular exercise and undivided attention in order to stay afloat. The swimmer gets a break from the worries and cares of everyday living. Concentrating totally on their senses and movement in the water, swimmers feel calm and relaxed after swimming.

Music, on the other hand has the power to move and stir emotions and instantly change our mood. A sad tune brings tears to our eyes and a cheerful rhythm makes us want to get up and dance. Perhaps man's fascination with rhythm allowed him to discover music. The first musical instrument invented was probably a drum. By combining rhythm and voice man discovered music. "It is not easy to determine the nature of music or why anyone should have a knowledge of it," said Aristotle about music. Pythagoras (550 BC) viewed music in mathematical terms, and he was the first musical numerologist who laid out the principals for acoustics. The Greeks discovered the correspondence between the pitch of a note and the length of a string. Confucius (551-479 BC) gave an important place to music in the service of a well-ordered moral universe. Music, he thought, revealed character through the six emotions that it can portray; sorrow, satisfaction, fear, anger, piety, and love. According to Confucius, great music is in harmony with the universe. Music in India was put into the service of religion in the earliest of times. Indian melodic ragas portray spontaneous rhythmic dialogues between narrations and instrumental sounds, and both are carried against insistent subtle beating of drums, giving Indian music a melodic excitement.

Music is considered to be a very pleasurable experience in almost all civilizations and cultures. Singing soothes the soul, and why not? Man was born with rhythm in his chest. A heart contracting and relaxing at regular intervals sustains his life. Regular intervals, a standard unit henceforth, applied to give meaning to time. Time became a working tool for mathematics and scientific understanding. A regular interval is a pulse, a rhythm in motion, a wave, a vibration, a beat. It must have been shortly after the discovery of music that humans moved to dance.

Dancing is one of the oldest of art forms and is found in every civilization and culture. It may be performed for a variety of motives, ceremonial, magical, theatrical, or purely aesthetic. Dancing is one of the most pleasurable experiences we know of. Even the medieval "Dance Of Death" is designed to alleviate pain by expressing feelings in movement. It is the coordination of movement and music that releases endorphins and alleviates emotional pain. One cannot dance without becoming happy. Dancing employs the senses of hearing and motion with rhythmic movement coordinated with music. Sensory excitation of neurons created by movement and sound causes the release of neurochemicals which instantly change the mood of a dancer. Dancing also helps to bring individuals closer to each other. This fulfils a deeper order of need by promoting an intellectual engagement with a prospective partner. It opens the opportunities for investigating the possibilities that might lead to fulfilling another important life preserving need, the survival of the species. Dancing also promotes self-expression. It is an artistic outlet by which a person can communicate with others. It fulfils a variety of sensory stimulations executed simultaneously, generating tremendous amounts of pleasure-stimulating endorphins.

Infants, as young as a few months old, start to move with rhythm and music. Babies try to sing as early as three months old. The baby has listened before it was born. As soon as the mechanisms of hearing are developed, the fetus hears and listens to its mother's heart beat and the sounds of the blood gushing in her blood vessels. Some behavior experts link man's fascination with the sound of crashing waves to the gushing sounds in mother's blood vessels that were first heard in the womb. They claim that walking along beaches is therapeutic and calming because it is a reminder of the feeling of security and warmth experienced as a fetus. Mothers sometimes place a ticking clock in the baby's crib to make their baby think mother is close by. This practice is also effective with kittens and puppies when they are taken away from their mothers. A ticking clock in their basket often calms them.

Some fathers like to believe that the unborn baby hears their voice too. Experiments were conducted during the sixties to teach the fetus to recognize its father's voice, and also to listen to music. Attempts have been made to teach babies in the womb many different things including the alphabet and counting. The results of these experiments are inconclusive.

All living organisms that have a nervous system are capable of producing neurochemicals that will make them feel good and experience pleasure. The mere transfer of electrochemical impulses through the nerves during the process of sensing causes the release of these neurochemicals which makes living beings experience pleasure. Humans have learned to increase their pleasure by participating in various activities that employ all of their senses. As we use our different senses the various centers in the brain controlling these senses also grow, increasing in size by branching out more dendrites, and we become capable of producing more neurochemicals. This will make us experience pleasure more readily. So the more active we are, the happier we will be. When we become more active not only does the brain become more capable of producing more neurochemicals, but all body systems, organs, muscles, and tissues develop, improving the performance of every cell.

In the next chapter we will discus the health benefits of exercise, and how by developing our muscles to receive their energy 100 percent from fat we reserve the blood sugar exclusively for the brain. When we maintain an uninterrupted energy supply to the brain, we will produce all the neurochemicals that are required to regulate all of our other body mechanisms, improving our health and fitness levels and strengthening our immune system as well.

Chapter 9

Physical Fitness and Exercise

Physical Fitness and Exercise

Exercise disrupts homeostasis, and speeds up all body mechanisms which must work harder to meet the demands for nutrients and oxygen required at the cellular level. The changes that occur in response to exercise are our body's attempt to reduce the stress that has been placed on its systems. By gradually increasing the intensity and the duration of the exercise on a regular basis, our muscles develop and grow in size, developing more mitochondria. Our cardiovascular system also develops to deliver the nutrients required by the body and minimize the stress imposed by exercise. Scientists have yet to discover how much exercise is too much or too little. It is up to us to decide how much stress our bodies can cope with. A gradual increase in intensity and duration is considered most beneficial. Many health scientists recommend twenty minutes of cardiovascular exercise three to four times a week to allow the body to develop to its potential and become fit.

To become fit means to develop our bodies to their fullest potential in order to meet the demands of everyday life. Exercise on a regular basis will develop our bodies to reach that potential. There are different levels of fitness a person can achieve. Few people push themselves hard enough to reach their maximum level of fitness. Most people are quite satisfied to become fit enough to do what they want to do.

There are four components to physical fitness and the four components must be met to allow a person to excel at their level of fitness. The four components of fitness are:

Flexibility - We must have flexibility to bend without injury to the muscles, tendons, ligaments and joints.

Strength - We need strength so that our muscles can work against resistance.

Muscle endurance - We need endurance so that our muscles can maintain physical effort over long periods of time without feeling fatigued.

Cardiovascular Endurance - Our cardiovascular system must be able to supply muscles with what they need and clean out the waste by-products of combustion in order to maintain homeostasis.

Regular aerobic exercise conditions our cardiovascular system. This is characterized by the increase of our total blood volume and the number of red blood cells which allows our blood to carry more oxygen. Our heart muscle becomes stronger and larger and each heart beat empties the heart chambers more completely, allowing our heart to pump more blood per beat. Our pulse rate, which represents the number of heart beats per minute, is lowered. Our breathing muscles become stronger, allowing our breathing to become deeper and increased volumes of air are inhaled and exhaled with each breath while the rate of breaths per minute is reduced. Our blood volume moves freely through our blood vessels because the muscles of our arteries contract and the movement of our skeletal muscles push the blood through our veins reducing our blood pressure.

Aerobic exercises include swimming, fast walking, jogging, fast bicycling, and playing soccer, hockey, basketball and cross-country skiing. Exercises that raise the heart rate for more than twenty minutes and use most of the major large muscles of the body such as the buttocks, legs, and abdomen, will benefit our cardio-vascular system the most.

Anaerobic exercises develop the strength and bulk of muscles. These exercises involve a sudden, all-out exertion of muscles lasting about 90 seconds during which time no fresh oxygen is consumed. Anaerobic exercises include sprinting, serving a tennis ball, and lifting weights.

People can shape up their bodies through exercise. To get an overall development of body muscles, one must participate in a variety of exercises. For example cycling will develop mainly the leg muscles, while playing tennis will develop the arms. Combining these exercises will ensure an overall balanced body. Incorporating a planned, regular exercise program, together with eating the nourishment that our bodies require, as well as allowing rest to heal and rejuvenate tired and injured cells, will promote a person's level of fitness. It is surprising how quickly fitness levels can excel by exercising about one hour three to four times a week, using all the muscles of our bodies.

Health Benefits of Exercise

Regular exercise invigorates and stimulates all our body mechanisms setting into motion an elaborate communication network that coordinates growth, differentiation, and the metabolism of the multitude of cells within our bodies. This communication takes place by direct cell to cell contact, and over long distances within our bodies. There are many hormones, pheromones, and neurotransmitters in our bodies, each designed to interrelate all aspects of the cellular processes of the various groups of our body cells. Hormones and neurochemical messages are released in our body fluids to be picked up by distant cells. Thus, all our body cells communicate with each other and are aware of what distant cells and organs are doing so that they may collectively continue the business of living.

Nerve endings in our muscles instruct muscles to contract and relax. The actions of muscles are deliberate, although perfecting our muscular movements seems a smooth and almost automatic action to us. We are aware of all our muscular activities when lifting, walking, running, or holding something. When our muscles contract or relax, they use energy by burning sugar or fat which are made up of carbon molecules. Burning a carbon molecule requires oxygen. When our muscles go into motion, all our body mechanisms go into action. Many hormones are released into our bloodstream, instructing our various organs to start releasing stored energy. Our body systems start to work to provide the oxygen and the nutrients to our muscles, and to remove the waste by-products of combustion. Our heart starts to pump faster and our blood pressure rises to allow our heart to pump more efficiently, our lungs expand more fully to allow more oxygen intake. Our liver starts to mobilize its glycogen. Fatty acids leave our fat cells and go to our muscles to be burned. This generates heat in our bodies. Temperature-regulating mechanisms come into action to cool our bodies when we overheat. Blood rushes to the surface of the skin, and activates our sweat glands, and cools us down by dissipating heat from the surface of our bodies. Our tiny blood vessels dilate and all the wastes from the extracellular fluids empty into the bloodstream. Our kidneys filter and cleanse our blood, our bodies get a good house cleaning, and our cells receive more oxygen and nutrients and we get rid of waste more quickly. Our performance level rises. Our internal environment becomes a better place for our body cells to prosper, and our rate of generating body heat becomes more efficient, raising our body metabolism as a whole.

Energy Use During Exercise

Regular exercise allows the body to initiate a multitude of physical changes. Regular exercise also causes the body's composition to change. Muscles learn to equip themselves with more fuel supply capacities, developing more muscle fiber in order to increase work capacity, and increase muscle efficiency for burning more fat. Hormones such as epinephrine and norepinephrine are released into the bloodstream, signaling various organs of the body to start releasing their stored energy. Fatty acids start to shed away from various fat deposits in the body and circulate freely in the blood stream where muscles can feast upon them and burn them for fuel. *During the first twenty minutes of exercise our bodies release the hormone epinephrine, which prohibits the level of insulin from rising in response to increased levels of blood glucose.*

During exercise, low levels of insulin allow fatty acids to be freely released into the bloodstream. Moderately strenuous exercise and an ample supply of oxygen allow a well-trained muscle to burn fat freely. Repeated aerobic exercise stimulates muscle cells to manufacture more mitochondria (that small organelle in the cell where burning of carbon molecules takes place, releasing energy). The heart and the lungs improve their capacity to deliver oxygen to the muscles, allowing a body that exercises regularly to become an efficient fat burning machine. Over a space of few weeks to a few months, depending on the person, the body can switch over to a fat burning metabolism through low intensity exercise lasting over twenty minutes, three or four times a week.

A simple exercise such as walking stimulates the muscles to pack their cells with the added mitochondria that in turn facilitate burning of more fat. Once the cardiovascular system reaches an efficiency rate that will deliver the required oxygen to the muscles, BINGO! There are all the ingredients necessary for muscles to burn fatty acids freely. After the exercise eases, our bodies continue to burn fat. Some evidence suggests that metabolism remains elevated by 25% up to three hours after intensive exercise, and fat may continue to be burned at 10% faster rate up to two days later (Whitney, Hamilton & Rolfes, 1990).

When our muscles become efficient fat burners, and receive their energy without disrupting blood sugar levels, then we will also enjoy a calm, more relaxed mood. We will be happier and enjoy life more, besides attaining an attractive physical figure. We will eat more regularly and not feel hungry for we can maintain steady blood sugar levels and an uninterrupted supply of fuel to our brain, producing all the neurochemicals that are required to regulate all of our other body mechanisms. Our immune system will also be improved by exercise.

The rate at which our bodies can utilize fat is dependent upon three major factors:

1- The availability of oxygen to our muscles. More oxygen is needed to break down a fat molecule than a sugar molecule. Fatty acid molecules must be broken down into two carbon molecules, and each cleavage requires oxygen. Glucose molecules have only one carbon molecule, therefore burning glucose requires less oxygen.

2- The development of mitochondria. The mitochondria are organelles in the cells that provide space for the combustion.

3- The presence of fuel (fat and/or glucose) to burn.

The key to burning fat is choosing a slow, steady, long-lasting exercise. This will achieve the desired effect: an improved capability of the lungs to take in more oxygen into the blood, and an improved capability of the heart to pump blood to the muscles more effectively.

People who smoke will always be inefficient fat burners. Their lungs are coated with smoke silt, and their oxygen intake capabilities tend to become limited. When smokers quit smoking they might gain a few extra pounds because they might replace the pleasure attained from smoking with pleasures attained from food (refer to the section on Nicotine, Chapter 3). Also, some research has found that nicotine increases the metabolic rate. When smokers stop nicotine inhalation, their metabolism will decrease and contribute to their weight gain. As soon as ex-smokers develop an exercise routine and discover the pleasures of exercise, their bodies will become efficient fat burners, and they will never have to worry about weight gain.

Chapter 10

Consequences of Dieting

Dieting To Lose Weight

When we start to diet and refrain from eating all the essential nutrients our bodies require, we place our bodies in crisis. We leave our body cells without the nutrients they require to carry out the functions necessary for living. This causes our bodies to take corrective measures to protect us from ourselves. Repeated shortages of nutrients prime the body to become susceptible to weight gain. We need to receive all the nutrients that our cells require to carry out our metabolic functions. When we restrict our food intake, the only option our bodies will have is to reduce our energy requirements by lowering metabolism. Lowered metabolism means that a person will be less active and burn fewer calories. Prolonged shortages of nutrients in our bodies cause many physical illnesses. Repeated failures to lose weight adversely affect our mental and psychological well-being.

Although dieting to lose weight has been accepted as a practice by dieticians and the medical profession for many years, many studies are indicating that very few people are able to lose weight and keep it off permanently through dieting as the so-called experts tell us. Most people who lose weight by restricting their diets eventually gain it all back and a little more. Repeated attempts to lose weight gradually render people much fatter then they originally were before they started to diet.

Studies were performed on wrestlers who practice fasting just before a wrestling meet (in an attempt to weigh less so they can compete in a lower weight category) and binge after weighing in. This study indicated that these wrestlers maintained a 14% lower metabolic rate than those who did not practice fasting (Steen, Oppleger & Brownell, 1988).

In another study, rats were placed on a yo-yo diet. Rats were fed a diet that made them become fat. Then the diet was restricted until the rats lost all the weight they had gained. The rats were fed again until they gained the same weight gained previously, then the diet was reduced again until they lost all the weight that they had gained. Sound familiar? The first time, the rats became fat in forty-six days and returned to normal in twenty-one days. The second time the rats became fat in fourteen days and required forty-six days to lose the extra weight (Brownell, Greenwood, Steller & Shreger, 1986).

These studies clearly indicate that repeated attempts to lose large quantities of weight lower the metabolic rate. *Two attempts to lose weight in rats made it twice as easy to gain weight, and three times as hard to lose it.* Think what a lifetime of yo-yo dieting can do to humans!

Chapter 10

Compulsive Eating

A compulsive eater will eat, indiscriminately, whatever he or she finds to eat and still not feel satisfied. This type of eating pattern usually starts after prolonged periods of food deprivation or weight loss. Many people develop reactionary behaviors to pull them out from stressful situations and often resort to eating compulsively when angry or emotionally unhappy and depressed. They shove food in their mouths without discrimination. After they diet most of the day, many people start to feel grouchy and depressed. They may suddenly decide to raid the fridge, eating everything in sight. (More about the emotional aspects of eating is found in Chapter 18.)

What we eat is what our cells will receive. What if we do not eat what our cells need? Usually there are reserves in our bodies that we draw from. We can manage to survive for a few days without doing much harm to ourselves. This is true for all nutrients except water, which we must drink (about ten glasses) daily. Without any water one cannot survive more than three days. Not drinking sufficient quantities of water over long periods of time can cause damage to the kidneys.

When we do not eat the nutrients required at the cellular level, we begin to experience sensations of hunger and cravings. These hunger feelings are an indication that our body needs nutrients and we will keep feeling hungry until we eat something.

When we decide to go on a diet to lose weight, we deliberately ignore hunger sensations. This is our attempt to exercise conscious control over our innate feelings of hunger. We resort to all kinds of ways to forget about our hunger and force ourselves to wait until it is time to eat. We regulate what we eat, when we eat, and how much. This totally disregards our sensations of hunger and cravings, and grossly interferes with and disrupts our bodies' innate mechanisms which control eating. Instead of reinforcing our innate mechanisms by seeking out the foods that may satisfy our hunger, reflecting and learning about our ourselves, the sensations we experience during eating, and the enjoyment we receive from meeting our needs, we start to resort to psychological mind games to control our hunger pangs. Instead of satisfying our hunger, we seek emotional and psychological help to train ourselves to control our hunger without eating. We even spend thousands and thousands of dollars attending weight loss clinics to learn visualization techniques and imagining ourselves becoming slim, trim, and supposedly sexy. One weight loss clinic provides its clients with magnetic stickers indicating how many pounds they have lost, and requests that these stickers be placed on their refrigerator doors to encourage them to refrain from eating. This clinic also advises their "fat" clients to place a full length mirror on the front of the refrigerator door so that when they open the refrigerator door to eat something, they first stop and look at themselves and remember that they became "fat" by eating.

When body cells are lacking a specific nutrient, the need for that nutrient does not diminish by visualization techniques or by looking in the mirror. As the body needs other nutrients, more sensations of hunger and cravings are triggered. Eventually a horde of hunger signals are triggered simultaneously, and sooner or later the person who is battling with his or her hunger succumbs and gives up dieting. Multiple signals demanding a variety of different nutrients will not allow dieters to consciously discriminate what they want to eat. They will start to eat anything and everything without discrimination, gobbling up whatever food they find, without listening to their bodies' specific requests.

Food Abuse and Eating Disorders

Eating disorders are groups of eating behaviors which have very serious consequences. Left untreated, these disorders can result in death. Eating disorders are common among young females around the ages of 14-25. They are much rarer in males. Unlike other illnesses, eating disorders stay with the person once they develop. The treatment of these disorders focuses on providing continuous emotional support and counselling, and fostering a supportive environment to build self-esteem and confidence. There are two distinct types of eating disorders.

Anorexia nervosa is a condition where the sufferer believes herself to be too fat even when she is extremely thin and emaciated. She abstains from eating and exercises excessively. The anorexia sufferer is always preoccupied with eating and weight problems, and tends to engage in aerobic exercises several hours a day to burn off calories.

Bulimia is a condition where the sufferer tries to vomit the food after an eating binge. The typical bulimia sufferer could be of average weight, very thin, or over-weight. Some bulimia suffers exhibit repeated attacks of pleurisy (an inflammation of the lining of the lungs, characterized by difficult, painful breathing, a dry cough, and sometimes a liquid build up in the chest), and /or hiatus hernia, caused by tightening of the thoracic muscles and diaphragm during self-induced vomiting.

One can suffer from both anorexia nervosa and bulimia simultaneously. Many who suffer from eating disorders are also known to abuse laxatives, amphetamines, or anything else that they think will help them in their attempt to lose weight. It is disturbing to know that a great number of people have demonstrated at least some of the symptoms described above at some point in their dieting careers.

Eating disorders are usually associated with low self-esteem, poor self-image, and a desire to exercise control over themselves and others. They exercise control over their body by starving it, and attempt to control their friends and family members by manipulating them to become concerned about them. They need to be the center of attention, where everyone around them is concerned about their health and eating problems. When adolescents become overly concerned and pre-occupied about their weight, fasting and food can become the most important things in their lives. They may start to drastically reduce their food intake and exercise for long periods of time. It is imperative that parents and friends watch out for these signs and seek help if their children or friends exhibit any of the above signs, to ensure they are not suffering from anorexia or bulimia. These behaviors are serious signs indicating the presence of some sort of an eating or other emotional disorder. Eating disorders are usually intertwined with emotional and psychological maladjustments. It is reassuring that not everyone who diets becomes anorexic or bulimic. It is also reassuring that if such disorders are diagnosed and treated early on, their prognoses become much more promising.

Chapter 11

War Against Fat People

A War Against Fat

Only in the past few decades has a slim, trim figure become fashionable. Before that, to be fat was associated with health, wealth, and beauty. The impressionist painters reflect this in their artwork. Paintings from the turn of the century show plump, full-figured maidens. The French painter Pierre-Auguste Renoir (1841-1919) painted nudes. His subjects were women who were full-figured and plump. By today's standards, women having such figures would be considered obese and unattractive.

There was a time when thin women were looked upon as sickly, and labelled as unable to bear children. People were afraid of tuberculosis, for it was the killer disease of the time, prior to the discovery of streptomycin and other drugs. A thin person was often suspected to be suffering from tuberculosis or other incurable illnesses which no one wished to be associated with. To be fat meant to be free from tuberculosis and other diseases. Ladies' fashions demanded padded hips, shoulders, bums, and busts to portray full figures, which were considered healthy and beautiful. Just think, in 1877, P.C. Duncan wrote a diet book on how to become fat!

Since the advent of the mass media, trendsetting advertisements, not to mention a cure for tuberculosis, slim and trim figures have become fashionable. Highly-paid, extremely thin model figures invaded the average home through the television screen. The same screen pressures the average TV viewer to change his or her eating habits for the worse with targeted advertisements. The population at large was implored to eat all sorts of goodies. People were enticed to eat ready-made foods saturated in fat and sugar, wrapped in convenient packages, and presented in the most appealing manner. Thin, sexy models used their sexuality to sell these products by implying that they attained their sex appeal by consuming the products they were selling. To look like these models became the desire of many women. The thin look was in and it was portrayed as sexy and beautiful, and full figures were portrayed to be ugly. Twiggy, a model from London became the top international model and lead a generation of women during the sixties to aspire to a figure like a twig. A thin, emaciated look became the fashion. This look is back again with a vengeance, despite the fact that we are still bombarded by advertisements imploring us to be part of a lifestyle which indulges in drinking beer and soda pop, and eating candy bars, potato chips, and doughnuts.

A raging war against body fat has been fought globally. Millions of people from every walk of life, pledge to lose every inch of body fat. They try all sorts of diets and fads to get rid of their fat. Americans spend billions of dollars each year on appetite suppressants and billions more on weight loss programs. Over half the

North American population wants to lose weight according to the Washington-based Food Marketing Institute. But there are more undernourished and yet overweight people in America today than any time in history. A 1994 Canadian Dietetic Association survey indicated that 80% of nine year-old girls have dieted to lose weight.

The consensus is that fat is ugly, and that fat people are lazy, unmotivated slobs. This leaves no choice to self-respecting people but to subject their bodies to brutal and cruel regimes. They try to lose weight, resorting to any means to get rid of their body fat.

The innocent casualties of this war are healthy young girls around the age of puberty. It is at this time that their hormones are adjusting and mobilizing their fat deposits within their bodies, enlarging their breasts, widening their hips and changing a young girl into a woman. This prepares them to become healthy women about to enter the most rewarding phase in their lives, getting ready for their child bearing years and motherhood. Young girls, and to some extent young boys, for they are also going through hormonal changes, are caught in the middle of a fat bashing war and are very vulnerable. Girls don't realize that once the change to womanhood takes place and their body matures, their bodies will self-adjust. The same thing goes for young boys. They grow fat, then lose it as they grow taller.

Of course there are some children who are more fat than others. There are many reasons why someone becomes fat. One reason for gaining weight during childhood and early adolescence can be attributed to hormonal imbalances, especially to low levels of thyroid hormone. Low levels of thyroid hormone can lead to lowered metabolic rate, and may cause depression. People with a low level of thyroid hormone will complain of feeling tired all the time and will have no ambition or energy to participate in physical activities. They will gain weight, their skin becomes dry, and in severe cases they lose their body hair. This condition is known as myxedema in older children and adults, and in younger children, juvenile myxedema. Low thyroid hormone levels interfere with the growth and development of a child. It is easily remedied by substituting the thyroid hormone externally. Parents concerned about their child's weight gain should consult with their doctor, or an endocrinologist to rule out thyroid and other hormonal imbalances.

When children are happy, active, and energetic and do not have any hormonal imbalances, parents should not be overly-concerned about their children's weight. Becoming overly-concerned about a child's weight and attempting to control what the child should eat or not eat, can rob the child from learning to seek his or her own food. Parents can help their children more when they introduce them to the taste of slow-release carbohydrates (see Chapter 19 Whole Grain Carbohydrate Source), and allow them to learn the taste of foods without the added fats and sugars. Let them learn how to cue into their sensory signals of hunger and satiation and eat only when they are hungry. By letting children enjoy their food and find pleasure when eating, and seek to find more pleasure by participating in other activities and sports, children soon develop all the skills they need to lead a healthy and happy lifestyle. Many chubby children grow out of their chubbiness as they grow older.

During puberty, reproductive hormones are released into the body. These hormones are released gradually in small quantities and are often irregular and sporadic early in puberty. Their release becomes more regular as the person becomes an adult. Reproductive hormones change the configuration of the body and this change reflects their irregular and sporadic release. There is a tremendous variation in energy expenditure during adolescence due to intense growth, especially if coupled with high activity. The total nutrient needs of the body are greater than at any other time in life, with the exception of pregnancy and lactation. A female's adolescent growth spurt begins at the age of 10 or 11 and peaks at around the age of 12. A male's growth spurt begins about the age of 12 or 13 and peaks about the age of 14. Any restriction of nutrients to the body during the period of growth throws the body into a crisis, slowing metabolism and priming the body to become susceptible to weight gain, which often continues into adulthood.

Adolescence is a time when young people become more aware of their physical bodies and selves. Rapid sporadic changes that occur normally are often perceived as becoming fat, so many young people start to skip meals and resort to dieting under pressure from the media and peers. There is no need for young people to subject their bodies to the atrocities of crash diets. Eating habits that are developed as teenagers and young adults have immediate and long term effects on health. This is the time for young people to develop good eating habits, and to expand on emotional, physical, and social levels.

When teaching adolescents about the changes occurring in their bodies during puberty, the subject of weight gain and dieting should also be elaborated. Educators should not hesitate to discuss weight problems in class. *Young people should be taught that restricting caloric intake lowers their metabolic rate and renders them more susceptible to weight gain.*

Parents and guardians can help the young teenager to enroll in recreational activities and sports teams to enrich and promote an active lifestyle. Teach children to do their activities to enjoy their lives and not to control their body weight. This is the time to expand and enlarge the basis from which the individual can learn to obtain joy from living. "Get off your butt and lose some weight" never works. When people are active, they release the endorphins that they require to stabilize and control their weight innately, and there will be no need for conscious weight controlling diets and regimes. In the enjoyment of life's little pleasures lies the ability to survive and overcome difficulties and hardships. During puberty, young adults are overwhelmed by the world they are about to enter. Their lives are about to change course and reach a more serious phase. Childhood games will be played for real. They will learn to fend for themselves. Those who are able to take up challenges, able to cope with stress, and are self-disciplined, they are the ones who can lead an active lifestyle, and know how to derive pleasure from everyday living. They will be the ones who will do well in life and remain healthy.

Chapter 12

The Experience Of Eating

How Our Relationship To Food Changes

We learn from our experiences with food. This learning process begins from the moment we are born. How we nurture our learning experiences with food greatly affects the development of our innate mechanisms which control eating.

Although the sucking reflex which is present at birth allows a baby to suck on the nipple, the baby quickly learns when it has had enough to eat. Babies indicate that they have had enough to eat when they push out the nipple with their tongue and smile, expressing their satisfaction. A mother always knows when her baby has had enough feeding. She will not be able to make the baby feed more. As babies grow and are introduced to solid foods, they encounter different tastes and various sensations that satisfy hunger. Children learn to seek out the foods that they have tasted before when they feel hungry.

Babies at about the age of six months have already learned how much formula they need to drink, and how long they need to suck mother's breast. Many breast fed babies experience the taste of the various foods that their mothers eat, because a mother's milk will taste like the foods she eats. Breast fed babies develop their selective eating skills sooner than bottle fed babies because a breast fed baby has already been introduced to various tastes and smells of the foods the mother has eaten.

Every encounter children have with food becomes a learning experience which is recalled when children feel hungry. Every previous experience with food becomes a menu of choice as to what children need to eat to satisfy their hunger. By experimenting with and experiencing the tastes, smells, and textures of various foods, children learn how to satisfy their hunger and gradually develop innate abilities to choose and eat according to their body's nutritional needs.

It is crucial that children develop good eating habits and learn to properly respond to their sensations of hunger, craving, and satiation. They should be encouraged to eat when they are hungry and recognize quickly when they reach the point of satiation, and not be asked to eat when they say they are feeling full. It is also important that they relate to their foods in terms of its tastes, smells, and texture. They should be allowed to request and clue into what they feel they need to eat. Parents should avoid the various practices they implement at the dinner table which promote and encourage emotional and non-nutritional reasons for eating. Innate eating skills are developed through eating practices aimed at satisfying hunger.

Human babies find pleasure in discovering their

abilities and becoming the center of attention. Often they use food to do so because it is there. Food is one of the first amenities easily attainable, so they start to experiment with it. Babies play with the food that is placed in front of them, they throw it about, squish it, spit it out, smear it on themselves and feed it to others. Babies learn by playing and they like to show off their accomplishments, they are generally seeking approval. "Look what I can do!" Parents find it amusing and encourage the infant to play with the food when they appear to enjoy the show. Children learn to play with food and it becomes a means of entertaining themselves and others at the dinner table. This is bound to have an effect on the child's relationship to food.

Mealtimes are crucial, since the child is learning about the taste and the smell of food, and how to satisfy hunger with food. The child often receives the wrong message. Perhaps he thinks that food is something to play with, and not just something to eat. Since everyone seemed amused to see his or her performance with food the first time he tossed it, the child will try it again. After a few performances, parents start to tell the child to stop playing with the food. All of a sudden the parents are not amused. The child becomes confused and perhaps thinks something is wrong with his food tossing technique. He may modify his technique in search of approval. And this time he gets yelled at and chastised for playing with the food. The poor baby cannot understand what is wrong, and becomes confused and hurt instead of learning about the food he is eating. He perhaps develops a dislike, maybe not a physical sensory dislike, but an emotional dislike, to the food he was playing with.

Many well-meaning parents use food to discipline their children by making them eat what is placed in front of them. If they refuse, they are punished or bribed. Have you noticed that most commotion, crying and temper tantrums occur around the dinner table? Good eating habits are developed by enjoying food. When children are upset during eating, they become confused about the foods they are eating.

Parents sometimes want to feed their child more, so they start to play games with the food. For example, parents pretend that food is an airplane, and the child's mouth is the hangar. Or they try to put a guilt trip on their children by coaxing them to eat for their grandmother's, grandfather's, or teddy's sake. Why should a child eat for his family's sake or his toy's sake? Why cannot everyone eat for their own sake? These actions confuse children, preventing them from learning about the foods they are eating.

Wise parents quietly remove the food and replace it with a toy when they see that the child is beginning to play with his food. Clowning and showing off can be accomplished with a toy.

Children are very honest. When they indicate that they do not feel hungry, they are generally telling the truth. They are much more in tune with their physical state of hunger and satiation than many adults. In Dr. Davis's experiment (Chapter 1) babies thrived on self-served diets and ate what their bodies needed. Even though they frowned and cried, they all ate salt. The little boy with the rickets, by his own initiative and without fail drank cod liver oil that was made available to him until his rickets had healed. He also drank all of his milk. That baby was able to recognize his need for vitamin A present in the cod liver oil and the calcium present in the milk. Of course, he did not know what he was drinking nor was he aware he had rickets. The taste of the cod liver oil tasted like what his body needed. In Dr. Fomon's experiment (Chapter 1), six month-old babies were able to regulate their dietary requirements. They drank more of the diluted formula and less of the concentrated formula. Children know when they are hungry and when they are not. They also know what to eat once they are familiarized with the taste of foods. The little children in Clara Davis's study (which has gained a lot of attention lately) demonstrated that children can make clear choices. During the first few days of the experiment, children sampled the foods, then began to make clear choices. They had specific preferences just as if they had a series of cravings for particular foods lasting for weeks at a time.

Children are also obliging. They will put up with considerable discomfort to please their parents and loved ones. They will force themselves to eat when they are not hungry to please or to avoid conflicts with their parents. This will disrupt and adulterate their innate mechanisms which control eating. It is much healthier and constructive to ask children what they want to eat, and when. If they are not hungry now they will ask for food when they are.

Mealtime can be a learning experience. New foods can be introduced and tasted, allowing children to feel free to taste and eat what they like. Children need to be exposed to various foods. Although children are equipped with inborn mechanisms to help them select their dietary requirements by triggering specific hunger and cravings, they must first learn by experiencing the various sensations associated with eating each food. The taste, smell and texture of their foods will have to be recorded into their memories so that they can develop an appetite for their tastes. Children who have never eaten carrots, do not know that the feeling experienced from the shortage of vitamin A can be satisfied by eating carrots. Children need to learn about the taste of carrots, their texture, color, and how carrots satisfy specific needs in their bodies, so that when the need arises in the body, for the nutrients found in carrots they will request carrots.

The atmosphere in which new foods are introduced to children is also very important. For example, when a new taste is experienced, their minds record in their memory the taste of the food, the texture, the color, the ambience, how it was presented, how they felt, how they were touched by their parents during dinner. When the mind recalls a food, the whole experience of eating that food is recalled, including all pleasant or unpleasant feelings experienced during the meal. This is referred to by scientists as **a conditioned emotional response.** Carlson (1991) describes conditioned emotional response as follows:

> *After having had pleasant or unpleasant experiences with particular objects, or with particular people, or in particular locations, we often experience emotional reactions when we again encounter these objects, people and places. If we had an unpleasant argument with someone, the sight of the person or the sound of his or her voice can produce some of the*

same reactions of the autonomic nervous system that occurred during the argument.

Adults entrusted to care for children should make a deliberate effort to ensure that all childhood experiences are pleasant and rewarding. Memories of past experiences are the reference files on which the child will rely in future decision-making processes.

To recognize what foods our bodies need, it is important that we eat when we feel hungry. If we impose food upon ourselves when we are not hungry, we will interfere with the development of our ability to identify what is needed by our bodies. When a child states that he or she is not hungry or has had enough to eat, it means that the child at that moment does not require nourishment. Why should the parents not trust the child? The child will later request a specific food he or she desires to eat. These specific requests draw upon very subtle, subconscious, instinctive knowledge of nutrients needed by the body at the cellular level. When children request specific foods, it is important that these foods are made available to them. Anything a child asks for is an indication of how that child is feeling, whether the feeling is one of physical nutritive needs or stems from psychological conditioning, parents should attend to the child's request. Parents should listen to what their child is saying and trust that their child is telling the truth. Unless the parent knows something else about the child's behavior, there is no reason to assume that the child is lying.

It is not wise for parents to impose their will upon a child and try to trick the child to eat food that he or she does not want. This will lead the child to develop an attitude toward the foods forced on him or her. The desire to eat, and a poor appetite are purely physical, although sometimes children learn to manipulate their parents much the same way their parents manipulated them when they made them eat food for reasons other than hunger. Children who refuse to eat can have many reasons for doing so. It could be that they are not hungry, or not feeling well, or they are allergic to the food they are pressured to eat.

Parents should remember that the dining table is not a place to teach a child discipline. Nor it is a place to test wills. It is a place to eat. By avoiding all confrontations with children who have problems with eating, the parent can find out more about what is bothering the child. Listening to children, trusting that children know how they feel, respecting children's wishes, and making every effort to meet their needs, will result in strengthening the relationship between parents and children.

Learning What To Eat

The mechanisms that trigger craving are complex. The hypothalamus houses the center which stores all nutrition related information and what is needed at the cell level (refer to Chapter 3, The Hypothalamus). All sensory messages from the tongue, the liver, the stomach, and the intestines terminate in the nucleus of the solitary tract. This nucleus processes information about nutrients that have been eaten and absorbed and conveys the information it receives into memory banks. When we need nutrients at the cellular level, we recall from previously learned tastes and experiences of foods that have succeeded before in satisfying our hunger, and bring them into consciousness as craving.

Dr. Gerald Bennett explains in his book "Eating Matters" (1988) that our feelings of hunger and satiation are conditioned reflexes and not conscious processes. We learn from each experience we have with food and expect the same response from that food when we encounter it again.

In an experiment, subjects were given soup and sandwiches for eight consecutive days. They were given a fixed amount of soup, and sandwiches cut into bite-sized portions, of which they could eat as many as they wished. There were two flavors of soup and each flavor had a different caloric content. One contained 25 calories per serving and the other contained 210 calories per serving. The subjects did not know the caloric value of the soups. These soups were served on alternate days. Subjects were allowed to have one serving of soup and take as many sandwiches as they wanted. At the end of eight days, it became evident that subjects were eating more sandwiches when the low calorie soup was served, and fewer sandwiches with the high calorie soup. Then the caloric value of the soups was switched, while their flavor and schedule remained the same, alternating daily. Subjects continued to consume sandwiches according to what they were accustomed to in the previous eight day period. This clearly indicates that we depend upon the learned taste, texture, flavor, and the way food satisfies our hunger, without knowing the caloric values of the foods we eat.

Of course, if subjects were to continue eating the low calorie soup and consume fewer sandwiches they would quickly switch to eating more sandwiches with the low calorie soup as their nutritive stores became depleted. Our innate mechanisms which trigger eating are not instantaneous, in that we do not, like magic, know what to eat, when to eat, and how much. Rather these innate eating mechanisms are developed through our experiences with food. What we innately learn about our food is also subject to modifications by which we constantly update and change the information we gather about our foods according to the experiences we encounter when eating.

We are constantly learning from our experiences with food and from the consequences of eating. We are also influenced by our parents and peers, by what we hear and what we see on TV about food. We associate food with status and class. We eat certain foods because of various customs and religious reasons. *But within the parameters of any culture, custom, or class, our bodies know what our nutritional needs are.* Learning to respond to internal cues of hunger and satiety, and eating the foods that we crave for, will result in meeting our nutritional needs. In many instances when we exercise control on what we eat and do not respond to our sensations of hunger, craving, and satiation, we end up eating everything else that we think we should eat and still turn around and eventually eat the foods we have craved for. Why not thoroughly enjoy ourselves and eat what we crave for in the first place? Why not develop our skills and recognize all our needs emotional or otherwise, and not develop habits of using food as rewards? Why teach our children to develop the habits of eating for reasons other than hunger, and attach non-nutritive values to the foods they eat? Why not develop our abilities and learn to respond to our physical sensations of hunger, cravings, and satiation?

Two studies were carried out by Birch and Marlin (1982) on the food preferences of two year-old children in a nursery school. In the first study, one group of children was given prune flavored milk as substitute for normal milk. The children were told that because they drank the prune milk they were being rewarded by viewing their favorite children's movie. The second group of children also drank prune flavored milk and were given the same movie to watch, but were not told that they were being rewarded for drinking the prune milk. After repeating this procedure eight times in two weeks, the children who drank prune milk for reward liked prune milk less than those who drank it without reward. Being bribed to drink prune milk made the children feel less favorable toward it.

In the second study, similar results were also obtained. Instead of a movie, praise was used as a reward. The children who were praised for drinking prune milk liked it less than those children who drank the prune milk, but were not praised. It seems that allowing children's taste buds decide their nutritional needs and what they enjoy is a far better way to motivate eating than bribes and praises. Frequently, parents encourage their children to eat the foods they are offered, and promise to give them their favorite dessert or a reward afterward. The child thinks, "the food must be yucky if I'm going to be rewarded for eating it". Bribing children to eat often puts them off.

Humans start recording experiences as soon as the brain is formed. Our sense of taste is fully formed at birth and changes very little afterwards. We accumulate various data about the tastes and the smells of food and how they satisfy our hunger. We store this information and refer to it constantly. Experiments indicate that six months after birth, babies can determine the nutritional content of their feeding. As we grow older we start to exercise control over our eating and undermine our sensations of hunger and satiation. We attach non-nutritive values to the foods we eat, and we eat for pleasure or because we are bored. These behaviors hinder the proper development of our innate abilities of craving and selecting foods according to our nutritional requirements at the cellular level, and we lose our ability to innately know the nutritional content of our meals.

Birch, McPhee, Steinberg, and Krehbeil (1986) showed the effects of "Clean Up Your Plate" practices. Praising or punishing children to eat what is dished out for them, makes them become less sensitive to the nutritional content of their meals. Their studies indicate that this kind of upbringing tends to weaken the body's physiological control mechanisms over eating.

Sensitivity to our nutritional needs can be gained back easily when we become responsive to innate requests of hunger and craving. By experimenting with our food like children do, we will rediscover the fun in eating. We will quickly regain our natural mechanisms by which we can innately learn to eat what we need to eat, when, and how much.

Chapter 13

Memory Storage

Remembering Our Experiences With Food

We are gifted with an inborn characteristic, the ability to learn from our experiences. We learn about our day to day dietary needs by making use of the information we learned in previous encounters with food. Our ability to innately learn about what we eat comes from our ability to sense the taste, smell, sight of the food we eat, how we chew and digest the food, and how foods affect our mood and well-being afterwards. Eating is a totally sensory experience and our mechanisms that control eating are all triggered and mediated through sensory messages. When we begin to relate to foods in terms other than what our bodies can sense and feel, we tend to distort our innate recognition of the foods that we eat.

The rate at which we forget something depends on many factors such as the conditions that were present at the time of learning, how often the information learned was recalled, and how meaningful the information was to the learner. We are able to learn more quickly and retain what we have learned longer if we associate the information to other things familiar to us.

The famous mnemonist S. could remember words, numbers, formulas, and could reproduce them many years later. He was studied by the Russian Psychologist Aleksander Luria (1968). S. also possessed a highly developed ability to perceive sounds as colors. This ability is termed synesthesia. S. could translate all spoken words into highly distinctive colorful visual images. He encoded all sound material seen or heard into structured collections of graphic images, and remembered them as a form of perception. Perceptual learning is the ability to learn to recognize stimuli that have been seen before and to distinguish them from similar stimuli. The primary function of this type of learning is the identification and categorization of objects and logic. S. was able to visualize sound in colorful images, therefore what he has heard was reinforced in two dimensions in the brain as colorful sight and also as sound. S. did not seem to forget anything he had ever learned. Although S. was born with remarkable skills, he spent a lot of time cultivating and improving his talent. Can we train ourselves to have the skills S. had? It is very doubtful that we could attain any of his abilities without the ability to interpret sound in graphic colorful images. Perhaps S. had a few neurons from his hearing senses reaching the center for vision, enabling him to see what he had heard (Refer to Chapter 4 Human Beings Are Sensory Creatures).

Learning from our experiences with food, although it is not exactly synesthesia, is a very powerful way of learning. We utilize all of our senses during eating. We see, taste, smell, touch and even listen to our food. Our bodies also record the post-ingestional effects of the food we eat and we remember how the foods affect us after we have eaten.

As we grow into adolescence we begin to think like scientists, becoming organized but flexible in the way we attack a problem. This flexibility in thinking enables the adolescent to compare situations as they actually are with situations as they might ideally be. We start to think of new possibilities. *During adolescence we become more aware of our physical body and become more concerned about how we look than how we feel.* We start to focus and experiment with new possibilities to improve our looks. We start to experiment with what we eat and begin to diet to sculpt our figure and become more attractive. It becomes very exciting to learn new ways to shape our bodies into the streamlined figures which are portrayed by the media as ideal. Television shows like "Fashion Television" where the average model is six feet tall and weighs 120 pounds are part of the reason many people start to sabotage their bodies in an attempt to look like the models on these shows, and render themselves susceptible to weight gain.

When our motivation is to have a model figure, we start to consciously control and interfere with our nutritional needs. We totally ignore the physical sensations and internal cues and requisitions, opting instead to take control of our mechanisms which control our eating. An egg for example, no longer is recognized by its taste and how much satisfaction we receive by eating it. An egg becomes a protein source, with 90 calories for a large egg, and 70 calories for a small one. An egg becomes a high cholesterol food to be avoided even when desired. A glass of orange juice becomes 75 mg vitamin C and is considered in terms of 120 calories sweetened, and 90 calories unsweetened.

The body cannot relate to orange juice as vitamin C, nor can the body relate to eggs as a collection of calories. Our mechanisms that control eating are far more subtle, sophisticated and efficient than that. Our "analytical" thinking proposes to us that we eat in order to sculpture the waistline, while our mechanisms which control eating are designed to select and choose foods which are required by our cells. Often our scientific thinking grossly interferes with and confuses our body mechanisms.

The brain stores all information, sensory or otherwise. Although it is convenient to think about storing information as a series of notes placed in a filing cabinet, experiences are not stored as concrete things but rather they change the way we perceive, perform, and think. They do so by physically changing the structure of the nervous system, altering neuronal circuits that allow us to perceive, perform, think, and plan. Therefore, the more an experience is repeated the more its circuitry is defined and implanted in our brain. This does not mean that once we learn something we are unable to change it. On the contrary, new information received updates the preexisting information and modifies and changes the brain circuitry accordingly. What happens when stored information is not reinforced, or the original information is only partially retained?

When we start to think about food in terms of calories and other data, we start to alter our sensory experience, with the taste, texture, and smell of the food. Our innate knowledge of relating to our food by sensory means becomes intertwined with academic and cognitive circuitry, such as calculating calories and remembering its protein and fat content, thus rerouting the information that we need to recall the food our bodies require at the cellular level. Our ability to recall the sensory experiences with foods according to taste, texture, flavor, and post-ingestional conditioning experiences, which are processed in the hypothalamus, becomes rerouted to the higher cognitive parts of the brain. Our mechanisms that control eating are governed mainly through various sensory impulses reaching the hypothalamus, therefore by changing the way we think about our food we weaken our mechanisms that control our hunger, craving, and satiation. Thus our recognition of the various foods by our sensory mechanisms is no longer acute enough to depend upon to select our bodies' requirements at the cellular level. We can no longer depend on our innate ability to select our own foods, and end up having to carry a calorie counter, protein value, and fat content booklet to check for ourselves what we may eat, instead of eating what our bodies *need and want*. Satisfying hunger no longer remains a sensory experience that will release endorphins so we may enjoy our eating experience, and develop our sensory eating skills. We are encumbered instead with the burden of having to calculate and measure and analyse the foods that we eat. Eating becomes an academic exercise.

The following experiment will demonstrate how we tend to change and distort our sensory experiences by mere suppositions and suggestions. Loftus (1975) showed a short film of a car accident to 150 students. She then divided this audience into two groups of 75. Students were asked 10 questions about what they had just witnessed. Subjects in one group were asked, "How fast was the white car going while traveling along the center of the road?" In the second group, students were asked "How fast was the white car going when it passed the barn while traveling along the country road?" In actuality, there was no barn shown in the film. A week later, subjects were asked another set of questions. One of the questions being, " Did you see the barn?" Seventeen per cent of the students who had been asked the question containing the false presupposition of the barn answered yes. Only three per cent of the subjects who had not heard the barn mentioned a week before responded affirmatively to seeing a barn.

For the same reasons, existing learned memories about food and eating can become distorted. When we start to clutter our minds with misleading information about the foods we eat, we begin to think about food in ways other than what our body can physically relate to. We tend to distort the information that we have about various foods that we have eaten. Being subjected to a false supposition once changed the perception of seventeen percent of the students above. Consider the constant bombardment of false information we receive about our food and nutrition several times a day throughout our lives, and you can imagine how much these false suppositions could distort our innate knowledge of the foods we eat.

We do not have control over the media and all those people who stand to profit from their suppositions. The least we can do for ourselves is relate to our food in terms of our sensory experiences with it, and discover the way in which food satisfies our feelings of hunger and produces feelings of satiation, and the pleasure we receive by eating.

When we start to think about an egg in terms of calories and cholesterol, we are bound to reroute our brain circuitry through other areas in the brain to calculate its caloric values, and focus on irrelevant information that our bodies cannot innately relate to. We ignore the fact that the body *can* relate to the precise memories and current experiences of taste, texture, smell, pleasure and satisfaction. By ignoring this, our ability to innately know what our bodies want becomes cloudy. Bits and pieces of information that we may recall are not sharp, not precise enough to depend upon to regulate our dietary intake to meet our dietary needs. Eating is a total sensory experience which is recorded in our memory, and we automatically and innately refer to it when we are hungry. We should not allow our innate knowledge of foods become distorted, vague, and misremembered.

Why would many of us think of an egg as calories, fat, or cholesterol? Why shouldn't we just enjoy eating an egg and remember how it satisfied our hunger? Why can't we trust ourselves? Why would we rather trust an expert? Our own bodies are the most magnificent experts and we are designed to spontaneously respond to all our physical and emotional needs. Why should we not respond to ourselves and our feelings?

Chapter 14

Biological Clocks

Life On Earth Has Natural Rhythms

All living systems upon this earth respond passively to the spinning of the earth upon its axis and around the sun. Life on earth is subjected to the predictable daily rhythms of light and temperature changes, and the changing of seasons. Likewise our physiological processes respond to the predictable cycles of Mother Earth. All our activities, including eating, sleeping, resting, and mating, are manifestations of our biological processes. These are activities that living organisms do every day and these activities are influenced by the regular cycles of day and night and the changing temperature of the earth. This rhythmic change in our world is reflected in rhythmic behavior of our biological systems which regulate our internal clocks. We have internal clocks that precisely time and schedule physiological events in all of our activities. Our internal clocks not only control the basal levels of our physiological systems, such as timing our sleep and wakefulness, feeding and drinking behaviors, thermoregulation, endocrine, renal, and reproductive functions, but they also influence the responsiveness of each system to the challenges that arise at different times of the day. Our internal clocks alert the appropriate homeostatic and regulatory mechanisms to become prepared to face these predictable challenges. This advanced preparation of our body mechanisms is crucial when synthesis of hormones and enzymes is required. Without advanced preparation, there would be delays of several hours in responding to the various demands of homeostatic corrections.

Therefore, our feelings of hunger do not just come about instantaneously because blood sugar levels are depleted, but rather because of an organized and timed sequence determined by our internal clocks preparing our bodies to meet their demands. By the time we become aware of our hunger our bodies have already been preparing our digestive system to ensure the availability of digestive juices, insulin and other hormones and enzymes for processing the food that is required by our bodies. Specific enzymes and hormones are already present in our system to digest and metabolize what we are about to eat. The idea of controlling what we eat is out of the picture. We must eat what our bodies are prepared to digest and assimilate. Otherwise we will not be in synchronization with our own bodies, and cannot expect our bodies to digest the foods that we have not prepared ourselves to receive. Eating our foods according to menus printed in books does not make any sense. It is important that we become innate eaters and reflect within ourselves to decide what our bodies have prepared for and what we need and want to eat. Our sensory messages will clue us into what our bodies' needs are and what foods our bodies are prepared to receive.

Many of us know what it feels like when we eat foods that are out of synchrony with what we normally eat at certain times of the day. For example, if we eat a high protein meal for breakfast we often feel tired and bloated until we digest it. We might feel dissatisfied if we eat cereal for supper. Of course if we train ourselves to eat steak dinners for breakfast and oatmeal for supper over a long period of time, we might gradually change our bodies' timing mechanisms to prepare different digestive juices and hormones to digest what we eat. Many people who work the night shift find it difficult to change their schedules to day schedules and they feel more comfortable eating oatmeal when they wake up at night to go to work, and prefer to eat foods high in proteins before going to sleep in the morning. Our bodies use energy when we are doing work, therefore eating a meal rich in carbohydrates before we start working will provide the energy we are about to expend. Our bodies also maintain and repair our cells and tissues when we are resting, so protein rich meals are needed to do this. A good protein and calcium rich meal is desirable before lying down to sleep.

Different people adjust to the rotational cycles of Mother Earth in their own way and their bodies prepare themselves according to the activities that they do. Some people consider themselves night owls and others consider themselves to be morning people. According to the activities to which they have accustomed themselves, their bodies learn to modify their internal clocks and prepare them to meet the challenges of their activities.

Our internal clocks are synchronized by the earth's revolving cycles and the activities we have to perform to secure our means of living during those cycles. Night predators, who have developed better skills to track their food at night, sleep during the day while other animals need daylight to find their way. However, when an organism is isolated form all environmental time cues; when light, temperature, food, and sounds are kept constant, the organism maintains its own independent timing to carry out its daily activities.

Researchers believe that the most important internal timekeeping mechanism is located in the hypothalamus. It consists of two clusters of nerve cells called the suprachiasmatic nuclei or SCN. Direct nerve fibers link the retina of the eyes to those clusters of nerve cells in the hypothalamus. When daylight light strikes the retina of the eye which has light sensitive neurons, the retina transmits light sensations to the SCN in the hypothalamus. The SCN in turn send impulses to other areas of the hypothalamus, to the pituitary and the pineal glands, and to other parts of the brain stem to indicate that it's time to wake up. These glands and nervous centers in turn send hormonal and neurochemical messages to other systems in our bodies, speeding up various organs and releasing insulin and other hormones to prepare our bodies to rise and go about our daily activities. When the day is done and light becomes dark, similar messages are transmitted in our bodies to slow down our physiological processes and we unwind, relax, and go to sleep. The heart, kidneys, adrenal gland, gastrointestinal tract, and the liver are all controlled by stimuli from the hypothalamus or the pituitary hormones which keep them in time with the rhythm of the day, instructing or stimulating various parts of our bodies to prepare for the various activities of the day.

Biological patterns associated to time of the day and the months were observed and documented as early as 400 BC by Greek philosophers. Aristotle noted the swelling of the ovaries of sea urchins at full moon. Herophylious of Alexandria noted variations of pulse rate during various hours of the day. Hippocrates noted a daily 24-hour fluctuation in his patients' symptoms. Ancient Greeks attributed the action of certain plants that opened their leaves during daylight hours and closed them at night to expressions of love to the Greek sun god, Helios. Plants which exhibit opening and clos- ing movements in relation to the sun are described to- day as heliotropic (Helio -sun, tropic -movement in the direction of.) It was believed that sunlight caused the plants to open their leaves and the absence of light made them fold.

In 1729, the French astronomer, Jean Jacques d'Ortous de Mairan conducted a simple experiment. He placed a heliotropic plant in a dark closet into which no light could enter, and observed it at various inter- vals. To his surprise, the leaves remained open during the daytime and closed during the night hours. This study was the first demonstration that indicated the existence of a biological clock, an internal mechanism that was capable of measuring time without external cues.

In 1832 a Swiss botanist, Augustine Paramus de Candela kept his plants *Mimosa pudica* (a plant whose leaves close and droop supposedly in response to light) under a continuous light source. He isolated his plants from sunlight and placed them instead in artificial light, with a series of six lamps burning at a steady intensity. He kept his Mimosas in constant twenty-four hour artificial lighting, which was equivalent to constant overcast sunlight. Candela found that the plants remained unperturbed and continued their cycle of folding their leaves and opening them. One factor had changed, the Mimosas shortened their cycle of opening and closing their leaves. The cycle lasted twenty-two and a half hours instead of twenty-four. This demonstration is referred to today as free-running. When freed from external environmental cues, an internal biological clock follows its own independent cycle.

Several hundred human beings were studied in various parts of the world during the first half of this century to examine the biological clock in people. These volunteers were deprived of all external cues that might indicate the time of the day. They were allowed to sleep, eat and function without the knowledge of time and in the absence of any cue that might indicate the time of the day to them, for periods of up to six months. All the human volunteers demonstrated that humans have a 25-hour clock (free run). When left to their own inner biological timing, human volunteers go to sleep one hour later every day, adding one extra hour each day to their previous day. Even though our biological clocks, when free-running, are on 25-hour cycles, we respond to and synchronize with the 24-hour day night cycle of Mother Earth.

Biological timing gives the organism the ability to measure its own time in an environment with fluctuating light and dark cycles and all the consequences of the earth's rotation. There are mechanisms in our bodies designed to maintain constant homeostatic conditions in the face of the changing external environment. These mechanisms have developed to predict and anticipate major and regular changes in the external environment and prepare their internal work schedule to meet the external changes.

There are several biological cycles. Circadian Rhythms are twenty-four hour cycles. Infradian Cycles (those cycles more than a day in length) can last for a month like the menstrual cycle in adult female primates, or a year, such as the annual rhythm by which deciduous trees shed their leaves. Cycles occurring once a year are referred to as Circannual Cycles and include hibernation in certain animals. Ultradian rhythms are cycles which are shorter than 24 hours and these include the heart and respiration rates.

Biological rhythms are very different from the Biorhythms you might find in the newspaper, alongside the horoscope section. Biorhythm does not constitute a science, and is based on an individual's birth date and forecasts horoscopes based on astrology.

The study of biological rhythms is a relatively new science. As late as the 1960's, scientists argued that de Mairan's phenomenon was not evidence that organisms had innate timing systems. It was argued that these cycles were not necessarily innate, but living animals and plants were perhaps affected by the earth's rotation, electromagnetic fields, or by cosmic radiation which served as cues that animals and plants used to sense or measure time. Researchers undertook to study the circadian rhythms of fruit flies, hamsters, and plants by taking them to the South Pole and placing their subjects on a turntable rotating counter to the earth's rotation. This way, as many external variations as possible were ruled out. All experiments continued to indicate the same rhythmic behavior that de Mairan first described.

Many studies have been carried out on various animals and plants, and each species seems to have a specific biological rhythm in a day when free-running. Flying squirrels have a 23-hour rhythm. Monkeys have a 24.5 hour day, and fruit flies a 22-hour rhythm. Many studies also indicate a genetic inheritance of biological rhythms.

Circadian Rhythms

The rhythmic cycle of biological timing of a 24 hour period is referred to as circadian rhythm (circa-from the Latin meaning about, dian-from the Latin dies, for days). Our bodies take cues from the levels of light and the temperature variations of the day. Our bodies may begin to measure time before birth. The fetus is believed to take its cue in its mother's womb according to the nutrients and hormones which regularly cross the placenta, and by her body temperature and activities that reflect her own circadian rhythm. (Newman, 1981).

The fetus receives cues about its internal day according to the mother's day. Babies continue to develop their own rhythm within the first few months after birth. As their circadian rhythm matures, infants develop a long nocturnal sleep period.

We learn to take our cues from other time signals

such as alarm clocks or even from the amount of deep sleep and rest we receive. Have you ever slept a deep sleep during an afternoon and woke up a few hours later feeling completely rested and thinking it was the next morning? Then you found out that you were out of synchronization with the rest of the world and it was nearly supper time and the day was not over yet? You likely bounced back to the earth's time and continued the day.

The eye plays a key role in synchronizing our innate timekeeping mechanisms to the day-length time of the earth's rotation. Blind people with damaged retinas can have unstable circadian rhythms. They experience uncontrollable nap-attacks. Stress and other psychological burdens can disrupt circadian rhythms of our bodies, alter our hormone secretions, and change our eating and sleeping patterns, de-synchronizing our internal time schedules. Changed work schedules, chemicals, insecticides, and other prescribed or non-prescribed medications that induce sleep or are stimulants, interfere with our bodies' rhythms and can disrupt the body's internal clock. Environmental conditions, including windowless work places, air travel, shift work, and all-night parties, all confuse our bodies's rhythms. Even the minor variation in weekend lifestyle confuses the circadian rhythms, with sleeping in on Saturday and Sunday being quite normal considering we have natural twenty-five hour cycles. But it is a rude awakening on Monday morning when we must return to the routine.

The shift of time of one hour each spring and fall between Daylight Savings Time and Standard Time often results in fatigue and requires more than a few days for our internal rhythms to adjust completely. Biological rhythms allow our bodies to schedule our physiological functions including establishment of sleep patterns, alertness levels, mood, and energy levels, synchronizing them with the outside environment. Biological rhythms dominate the whole spectrum of life processes, including fertility, sexuality, eating, drinking, metabolism, mood and behavior, skin, bone, and muscle development, aging, and even the time of our death.

Hunger and Circadian Rhythms

Our innate functions become synchronized with the external cycles of light and dark, and are cued to the time of the day to allow our bodies time to sleep and to be alert, to eat and to digest. Our bodies organize and arrange our life's functions to coordinate and prepare our physiological mechanisms to meet our needs, according to the various times of the day, as to when it is best to perform each and every biological function.

We have become accustomed to eating three meals a day and snacks in between. A person who takes lunch breaks at twelve noon every day develops a habit of eating regularly at noon and this person will regularly feel hungry at that time. Some people will feel hunger pangs at their regular meal time. However, hunger is not solely dependent on the time elapsed since the last meal. This is clearly illustrated in the daily eating habits of people who volunteered for experimental studies and spent days alone in enclosed windowless rooms completely isolated. Their meal times staggered once they no longer were able to cue in to the earth's rotation time. The time between waking up and breakfast stretched to between six and eight hours, the time between breakfast and lunch stretched eight to ten hours, between lunch and dinner was about ten to eleven hours (Aschoff, 1986). This clearly indicates that our eating behavior is controlled by a twenty-four hour schedule synchronized by the day and night cycles of the rotation of the earth. Our body takes its cues from the day-length time to prepare its digestive juices and at noon we feel hungry.

The hunger we experience at 12 o'clock noon is a form of habit rather than a true indication of the body's need for nutrients. Our physiological systems prepare themselves according to the activities that we have become accustomed to performing regularly. Our bodies prepare digestive juices and hormones to meet the challenges of what we are about to do so they can efficiently and quickly deal with habitual food intake at certain times of the day.

Jane Hyman Wegscheidre in her book "The Light Book"(1990) explains that before it grows light each day and we are awakened, the heart rate, the blood pressure, and body temperature start to rise. By about 5 a.m., the levels of the hormones cortisol, insulin, and other peptides start to increase in the blood to help us defend against the stresses that we will encounter as we meet our daily activities. The hormones and digestive juices released give us an appetite for high carbohydrates. Noradrenaline levels start to increase at about 9 a.m., raising energy levels and mental alertness. This time is more conducive for decision making. Our body temperature continues to rise, and by 12 noon it peaks.

Many studies indicate that the level of alertness and the metabolic rate take a dip for one hour or so after lunch, justifying a siesta, then rise again towards the afternoon. Our blood pressure peaks at 3 p.m., and by 5 p.m. body temperature begins to fall. At about 6 p.m. after our evening meal, serotonin levels increase and muscles begin to relax. Mental activities such as studying, learning, and reading undertaken at this time increase the levels of serotonin causing our muscles to relax further. By 10 p.m. blood pressure falls, heart and metabolic rates decrease, helping the individual to get ready for sleep. At about midnight or so growth hormone levels rise and during sleep our bodies repair cellular damage sustained during the day. Individuals who stay awake all night find that their lowest performance is around 3 a.m. to 5 a.m.. Performance starts to improve around 6 a.m. even in subjects who have been kept awake all night. Many night shift workers and individuals who party all night have reported new vigor experienced at dawn when daylight strikes the retina of the eye and excites our suprachiasmatic nucleus in the hypothalamus, calling all our body mechanisms to rise and meet yet another day.

People should not feel guilty when they get up at night to raid the refrigerator because they are hungry. When someone feels hungry in the middle of the night, it must be protein or calcium their body is calling for to do its repair work. Perhaps that is why many people tend to crave for a glass of milk to help them go back to sleep. Perhaps this is part of the reason why pizza restaurants do brisk business between the hours of eleven at night and one in the morning.

Chapter 15

The Challenges We Face

The Joy Of Living Is In The Challenges We Face

Our well-being, both on emotional and physical levels, is directly related to the performance of our day to day activities. The more active we become the happier we will be and the more our whole body will develop.

When we do not employ our abilities we lose them. For example, when we do not exercise muscles, the muscles atrophy and shrink. When we do not use reading or writing skills they can be forgotten. All our physiological processes must remain active so they continue to grow. In this world of ours nothing stays the same. When we think we are holding our own, time is changing. Nothing remains unchanged. If we are not growing we are dying.

There are times in our lives when we feel good about ourselves and have more self-confidence, feel more cheerful and energetic, and experience a feeling of vitality so intense we almost tingle feeling happy. There are other times we do not feel so happy. We experience various levels of happiness. The degree of happiness we experience is directly related to the amounts of endorphins we produce.

The happy feelings that we often experience are an indication that our body cells are in a state of contentment. If there have been enough endorphins and neurochemicals released to effectively calm and restore the internal environment, then the needs of our body cells have been met. When we feel unhappy, it is an indication that we need to change something in our lives, in some way or another, to regain the state of happiness which we experienced before. We need to find ways to feel better, and search for better ways to relate to the environment and the conditions around us. We start to think in terms of changing our relationship with the world around us, in an attempt to improve the world within us. We don't always do this, though, and this is when we start to have problems.

Our feelings indicate to us what our needs are. When we do not feel good, to make us feel better we sometimes decide to take a breather and go away. We decide to go to the movies, perhaps pursue a hobby, join a club, join a swimming program, play ball, call a friend, order a pizza or eat something that we want (perhaps chocolates?). These changes often work and we feel better. Getting out of a routine and doing something new or different, becomes more fulfilling, and makes us feel better. By doing something different and interesting we soon begin to produce the neurochemicals we need to get rid of the blues.

At the miraculous moment of birth each one of us entered the world carrying a distinctive set of capabilities, totally ignorant, knowing not what the future held for us, or indeed, even that there was such a thing as future. Everything we achieve in this world is through learning. We learn how to overcome inner feelings of grief, pain, fear, anguish, despair, guilt, loneliness, and sorrow that we often experience. We learn to replace them with courage, wisdom, hope, forgiveness and love. The miracles in life lie in our ability to learn and change the way we perceive, act, and feel. We learn that we can overcome the feelings of sadness or despair, and replace them with joy. Our feelings guide us through the learning process. Our feelings guide us every step of the way. They help us realize that we can improve our lot and overcome all negative feelings by our actions and hard work. We begin to recognize a potential within us that helps us grow emotionally and we can rise above our problems and face up to the challenges in our life. We learn to apply our inherited capabilities wisely, and through persistent effort, we can enhance our lives and the lives of others around us.

Most physical and emotional problems arise when we do not utilize our capabilities. Many of us think that we are not capable. Sometimes we do not even bother to take stock of what we have. We tend to dwell on our disabilities, or perhaps think that this is a cruel world and we wallow in misery. We must remember that life is not easy. Nobody has it easy. We all have to learn to crawl, stand up, walk, and then run. We had to learn every painful little detail in every stage of our progression, and for each time we learn something, our bodies release serotonin and other neurochemicals that will make our learning experiences worthwhile. For each accomplishment, and every little thing that we learn, we are rewarded with feelings of happiness and joy. The magic of living is found in discovering our abilities, and our strengths, and in overcoming difficulties in our lives. It is not what we have inherited in our genes that makes us feel good about ourselves, but rather it is what we do that determines our happiness, health, and fitness and makes us receive fulfilment from living.

Chapter 16

Maximizing Our Capabilities

Maximizing Our Capabilities

Our feelings and sensations hold the key to our abilities and accomplishments. Through our ability to feel we are able to learn and know all about our world and ourselves. It is our ability to feel pain that protects us from dangerous circumstances and our ability to experience pleasure that compels us to pursue learning and discovering more about ourselves and the world we live in. Thus through learning and experiencing pleasure, we are able to change and reach a higher level of understanding of ourselves and our environment.

We enter this world with a blueprint of characteristics that are passed on to us from our parents. We each carry a specific set of genes, which determine all of the characteristics that we could potentially have. These characteristics are developed afterwards, according to our life experiences. Despite what we inherit from our mothers and fathers, we enhance or detract from our genetic blueprint by the way we lead our lives. Everything that we do during our lifetime either maximizes or takes away from the gift package that we have inherited at birth. For example our sense of taste is genetic. It is fully formed at birth and changes very little afterwards. It is how we use our gift of taste that decides our sensitivity and ability to benefit from this gift. Everything that we do is subject to modifications throughout life. These modifications come about according to how we interact with the external world around us, and what we can learn from these interactions. We often learn to become insensitive to our feelings. In many instances we tend to confuse our thought processes by attaching non-nutritive values to the foods we eat. We learn to ignore our sensations of hunger, craving, and satiation. This often results in losing our abilities to select the nutrients our bodies require. An undernourished body leads to an undernourished mind, placing all our capabilities in jeopardy.

We do not have to do much to attain health, fitness, and happiness. All we need to do is to be responsive to our feelings and sensations. These feelings and sensations are the only way our bodies can communicate with us about our internal conditions and needs. When we respond to our sensory messages, we feel great. We experience positive, lively, energetic feelings after meeting our bodily needs. When we do not respond to our needs, our endorphin levels drop and we do not enjoy our lives as much as we are designed to do. When too many excitatory messages are emitted and we ignore their signals, we throw a tremendous stress on our bodies and our needs will not be met. For example, if we do not drink when we feel thirsty, we probably will feel very tired and dry. If we continue our state of thirst for too long we can damage our kidneys and perhaps die. If we sit around in the house all day, moping and groping, refraining from doing exciting activities in which we will learn something new and different, the level of neurochemicals released by the brain is lowered, and soon we will feel depressed and might even think that life is not worth living. All the sensations we feel, whether pain, thirst, hunger, or others, are triggered whenever our internal world needs to interact with the external world to meet our needs. When we solve the problem, and our needs are met, we release neurochemicals and we feel good.

Parents have an obligation toward their children to raise them without allowing them to lose the gifts they were born with. What would have happened to Mozart or Albert Einstein if their genius was suppressed? We owe it to ourselves to nurture and attend to our feelings, physical sensations, and thoughts. Our feelings, sensations and thoughts are designed to bring out the genius in our genes. The human body is designed to sense and guide itself to do what is good for its existence. We know what is good for us, and what will enhance and elevate our bodies and our minds.

The human body is designed to enjoy living. The autonomic nervous system has mechanisms in place that are triggered subconsciously to inform our conscious mind to undertake that which is required so we continue living and enjoying our lives. The release of two types of neurochemicals in the body, excitatory and inhibitory, serve us well. Excitatory chemicals instigate the need for change by triggering various sensations that will inform us about specific needs. Inhibitory neurochemicals are released in our bodies after we have satisfied the requests, and our internal environment is stabilized. For example, when there is a shortage of water in our bodies we feel thirsty and are thus compelled to drink. When our energy reserves are down, we feel tired and we are compelled to rest. When our bodies are short of nutrients, we feel hungry and we eat. We have an internal clock that regulates when to sleep and when to be awake. Excitatory neurochemicals instigate these feelings. Often we take our cues from our inner conditions and do what is necessary to provide a comfortable environment for us to live in. When the tasks are done, inhibitory neurochemicals are released and we feel refreshed, satisfied, and happy. The inhibitory neurochemicals also counteract pain. The design of our bodies is such that the sum of all our living experiences is reflected in our mood, which is set by the various neurochemicals that are released into our bodies by the process of living. Thus we develop an inner intelligence which is aware of what we need to do in our lives to enhance our health and well-being physically and emotionally.

Indulgence

We may think that human needs are vast and endless. We might think it is a tall order to meet all our needs. However, it is not our needs but rather our desires that are vast and endless. Basic human needs are simple and straightforward. They are the basic needs of survival. We are designed to ensure the survival of every cell of our body by maintaining homeostasis. The homeostatic conditions are monitored on a continuous basis and specific hormones and neurochemicals are triggered automatically to regulate and adjust our internal environment. Each change in the homeostatic condition triggers the release of a certain chemical that is somehow translated into a feeling which is designed to prompt us to recognize and deliver to ourselves the necessary nourishment or whatever else that we must do so our body cells can continue living.

When we meet our basic survival needs, we experience pleasure, which awakens a yearning within us to attain more fulfilment from living and experience more pleasures. We explore the various ways that we have learned to increase our pleasurable experiences. We start to indulge, experiment, and explore in activities that will increase the rush of endorphins into our system. We begin to overdo things that give us joy and pleasure. Sometimes, sooner than we realize, we get carried away. We overeat, over drink, overindulge in smoking and other activities that give us pleasure. Depending on what sort of experience we indulge ourselves in, we develop certain habits and certain ways of boosting our endorphins. *Sometimes we neglect to take our cues from our internal sensations and feelings, and release our tensions and anxieties by resorting to habits we have learned which will give us a rush of endorphins that make us feel good.*

Throughout history there were always cultural teachings which constantly warned us against our pleasure-seeking instincts so that we might be saved from our overindulgence. Thus, pleasure-seeking was often regarded as immoral and sinful. There is a fine line between the pleasures we seek to satisfy our needs and the pleasures we receive from overindulging.

The pleasures we experience from meeting our needs are uplifting and refreshing, while the pleasures we experience from overindulgence can, and often do become uncontrollable. Pleasures we receive by meeting our needs give us feelings of contentment and satisfaction, and the pleasures we receive from overindulgence lead to feelings of excitement. One might also say that the pleasure we experience from overindulgence can become compulsive and addictive. As we recall from Chapter 4, addiction is the result of neurons developing tolerance to repeated excitatory stimuli caused by drugs. Becoming addicted to something does not necessarily mean that there is some external substance that we must consume and abuse. People become addicted to doing crossword puzzles, or playing video games, or gambling, and many other circumstances where their aim is to receive gratification through scoring points. They stop doing things to learn from them and enhance their physical and emotional well-being, but rather do them to seek excitement to gratify psychological needs and self-worth. There are people who are addicted to exercise and building body muscle to the point where they neglect everything else in life, to receive physical and psychological gratification from building up strong huge muscles.

Many of us know where to draw the line and recognize when we are about to cross the border and indulge ourselves in something more than just enjoying ourselves and learning from our experience. We are very careful not to cross that fine line when participating in activities that have the reputation of having addictive consequences, such as alcohol consumption, or gambling. Many people for instance watch out when they are consuming alcohol. They reflect within themselves to check on how they are feeling after the first or the second glass of wine or beer before they take another drink. Gamblers who are doing it for fun check their pocketbook and realize it's time to quit. These people are not necessarily afraid of becoming alcoholics or compulsive gamblers. To become an addict there are many other components. The point is that when we pay attention to our actions, we know and recognize the fine line between having fun and getting carried away, developing habits that give us gratification without improving our lives. If we watch out for ourselves and take our cues from how we feel in everything we do, we will always recognize and know when we are crossing the line. Although certain habits cause the release of specific neurochemicals which will allow us to experience pleasure, habitual indulgence in these activities will eventually lead to relying on these habits as the main source of our pleasure. *The physiological and biological functions of our bodies are based on our ability to receive pleasure in all the activities that enhance our living conditions so we may continue to participate in life-promoting and enhancing activities.*

In Chapter 3 we talked about how the structures of the brain cells change in the various centers of the brain according to the activities we pursue, and different neurochemicals are released by doing different activities. For example, the excitation of the center for taste produces serotonin. Lovemaking produces dopamine. Stimulation of the nerve endings found under the surface of the skin causes the release of enkephalin which alleviates pain and discomfort. There are likely many other neurochemicals that have not yet been identified. When we are indulging in one activity, we receive sufficient endorphins from that activity and feel satisfied. We may therefore tend to neglect other sources of endorphin-producing activities.

To make our lives full, wholesome, and satisfying, we need a variety of these neurochemicals that give us pleasure by elevating our spirit, reducing our pain and maintaining a good mood. Humans experience a variety of feelings and moods (as studied by Dr. B. Lyman, discussed in Chapter 5: Human Beings are Sensory Creatures). We need to experience all the various sensations and moods, and not short-change ourselves from the full potential of pleasures that we could receive. Our physical, emotional, and spiritual growth is derived from and developed by the variety of our experiences. A variety of emotional feelings cannot be brought about through indulgence in one type of activity, and the production of one neurochemical, from one center of the brain. We need to have all the various neurochemicals that give us all the different feelings and moods. We need to capture the soft and the vibrant, the wholesome and the triumphant moments of our lives. We need to experience all the effects of all the various activities that modify our mood naturally as a result of our actions and thoughts, so we may truly express ourselves in our own different and unique style. Each different feeling and mood we feel as a result of our effort unleashes and opens our minds to a better understanding of ourselves and our world. We grow through our experiences and learn to face and over-come adversity by using what we have learned. To main-tain well-balanced physical and emotional fitness, and strengthen the body's immune system, we need to bal-ance the various neurochemicals released into our bod-ies as a result of our own efforts and actions. We can make our lives meaningful and complete.

Chapter 17

The Dilemma of Weight Gain

The Dilemma Of Weight Gain

Besides many people's beliefs that obesity is hereditary, and that there are genetic factors which determine the number of fat cells in the body, we cannot ignore the major role metabolic factors have in obesity. Although there are differences in metabolic efficiency between a fat person and a thin person, many of these differences are brought about by exercising academic control over eating. The latest findings indicate that the number of people deemed overweight in North America has increased from 25% in 1982 to 33% in 1993, despite the North American obsession with weight control and the healthy eating craze. According to the Washington-based Food Marketing Institute more than 60% of shoppers have made changes in their food regimen in the past decade, with the desire to lose weight being the number one health concern driving those changes. What is most interesting is that all these genetic and other physiological factors have always existed, yet never before have we been so academically knowledgeable about the foods that we eat. Never before have we been so keen to practice our academic knowledge about healthy eating. Still, the number of overweight people is increasing. This tells us that the problem is not entirely dependent on what we eat or on our genetic make-up but rather, the problems of gaining weight lie in exercising academic control over eating.

During the past few decades, a multi-billion dollar diet industry has been thriving. Almost every man, woman, and child has become obsessed with exercising control over his or her eating, which grossly undermines our bodies' metabolism and our innate mechanisms that control eating, and renders us totally insensitive to our feelings of hunger, craving and satiation.

It is evident from the continuing increase in the number of overweight people, that diets and other weight management programs are not working. Kramer, Jeffery, Forster, and Snell (1989) reported that five years after participating in a fifteen week behavior modification program for excessive eating, only three per cent were able to maintain the weight loss they achieved. Ninety-seven percent had returned to their original weight after four to five years. Some even gained more weight than what they had originally started with.

There are many factors that cause a person to become fat. Scientists have discovered several proteins that are believed to control the deposits of fat in our bodies. Knoll (1982) isolated an appetite suppressing protein from human blood and named it Satietin. Harris, Bruch, and Martin (1989) extracted a protein from the fat cells of rats, that inhibits the growth of fat cells. Other scientists were able to identify a gene that determines the number of fat cells in the body. Although these discoveries indicate that there are mechanisms that control the deposit of fat in fat cells, what triggers these mechanisms is not well known.

Scientific research agrees that the reason for weight gain is multifactorial. It includes many physiological, social, and environmental factors that encourage overeating. For example, children are often praised or punished for eating or not eating what is put in front of them. Adults are influenced by their desire to become thin and they reduce their nutritional intake. These behaviors tend to suppress and disrupt our innate mechanisms that control eating.

Our bodies have profound neurochemical signaling mechanisms which ultimately control hunger and satiety. These mechanisms develop through our experiences with food. We strengthen our ability to innately balance our energy intake to energy output when we become responsive to our feelings and take our cues from within as to how we feel and what we crave to eat. Losing weight becomes monumentally difficult without employing our bodies' innate and selective eating and satiation mechanisms.

Almost all weight loss programs focus attention on restriction of food intake. These programs throw tremendous stress on our bodies and render us insensitive to our feelings of hunger and cravings. They teach us to carry a calorie counter and a calculator and ultimately count and calculate everything we eat, note every speck of food that enters our mouths, weigh and analyse its fat, protein, and carbohydrate contents, determine its cholesterol, vitamin, and mineral contents. This style of eating robs from us the sheer enjoyment of eating and relating to our food in terms of our sensory experiences with it. The delightful sensation of eating and choosing what our bodies need can be a sensuous, exhilarating experience that we should not deny ourselves. It reinforces and strengthens our ability to become selective eaters, able to respond to our nutritional needs at the cellular level.

Our obsession with losing weight has turned us into calorie counting freaks. We count the calories we eat and the calories we expend. There are lengthy charts indicating how many calories each activity will burn. For example jogging will burn 400 calories per hour, swimming burns 350 calories per hour. Sitting idle and not doing anything burns 60 calories per hour. Love-making will burn 300 calories (one cannot help but wonder if that is with orgasm or without, and how they arrived at the figure in the first place). Some joggers have confessed that when they run they think about the calories they burn with every stride they take. It motivates them to continue the struggle to burn those extra calories.

By using calories as a motivation for physical activity, we have been robbed from the enjoyment we could have received from the sheer pleasure of participating in these activities. When people are exercising merely to burn calories and they are not enjoying themselves, they can get injured and still continue to suffer the pain for the sake of burning calories and losing weight. When people are not enjoying what they are doing, they will most likely not continue their activity after they reach their goal of losing the weight they want, the result of which will be that they soon will start to gain back the weight they lost. When we are doing any activity, whether it is eating or exercising, we should enjoy what we are doing. Perhaps diets do not work because restricting our food is not fun. Consider the other side of the coin: exercising is no fun when one is hungry or half starved.

The Quest To Lose Weight

The amount of fat that we can burn is totally controlled by our innate metabolic functions. The idea of controlling body weight *at will* is a false expectation. What is possible on the other hand, is to ensure that we allow ourselves to find pleasure in all the things that we do including finding joy and pleasure in eating. When we are enjoying what we are eating, we can be sure that we are receiving all the proper nourishment required by our bodies.

All our metabolic reactions including the burning of fat, are innately controlled. We have no control over our body mechanisms. Our bodies innately decide when to burn fat and when to store it. Rationing our food to force our bodies to burn fat causes us to become fat in the long run. People who control their weight by restricting their diet remain in a constant battle with themselves. There is a constant tug of war between our will to control weight, and our bodies compensating for the rationed nutritional intake by lowering our metabolic rate. *We should never be at war with ourselves!* There is no need for this constant external control to regulate body fat content. Once we give up external control over weight management, our bodies will do a better job managing our own ideal weight.

Our bodies are designed to inform us of our requirements. Our hunger and cravings and sensations of satiety, are designed to inform us as to what we need to eat. Our feelings are manifestations that allow us to know and recognize what it is that we must do to keep ourselves fit and healthy. *The indication that we are achieving our objectives and eating the right nutrients is conveyed to us by experiencing pleasure and joy.*

Attaining A Slim Trim Figure

Our experiences in life can be very rewarding and successful when we join forces with our natural abilities and maximize the gifts bestowed upon us at birth. The well-being of the physical, emotional, and cognitive aspects of our lives are dependent on how we conduct ourselves and enhance our inborn capabilities, how much joy and pleasure we experience, and the amount of endorphins we produce.

Losing weight through restricting dietary intake will not last. We must work with the body's natural abilities. Starving ourselves is unnatural. All those who lose weight through dieting will inevitably gain their weight back and a little more once they can no longer endure starvation.

We must work with our bodies and not against them. We must care for the well-being and the survival of each cell in our bodies. We must respond to every need made known to us through our feelings. We must aim to find satisfaction, contentment, and joy in everything that we do and think about. We must find our answers from within ourselves and respond to our sensations and feelings. By doing that which makes us feel good we can live long, prosperous, happy, and healthy lives, and a slim, trim figure will be a spin-off benefit of a healthy lifestyle.

Chapter 18

Emotional Feelings

Emotions Control Our Lives

We relate to ourselves and other people, as well as animals and objects, in terms of how we perceive them and the information we have about them. Our relationships are very often influenced by our mood and how we feel. Our opinions are, at first, based upon how we feel, but gradually as we grow older and learn to think and make judgments, our opinions become based on our perceptions in light of what we have learned. Much of what we learn is very often influenced by how we feel.

All sensations, whether pleasant or painful, experienced momentarily or recalled from the past, cause the release of neurochemicals which determine our mood. Once we perform an activity and we enjoy it, the neurochemicals released from that activity compel us to repeat the activity again and again. We like the good feelings generated from that activity and are eager to repeat all activities that give us pleasure. We sometimes put up with discomfort and pain if we think the rewards will give us delayed pleasure. For example, when we start to exercise we develop pain in our muscles from lactic acid build-up, but our desire to look and feel good allows us to put up with discomfort now for greater rewards later.

Our habits are formed according to the activities that give us pleasure. Whenever we encounter a negative or painful feeling, or the memory of a painful event in our lives, we quickly resort to the thing that we know will release endorphins, making us feel better. A common, easy, and rewarding act that will release serotonin instantly into our system is eating sweets and desserts. Many of us have been conditioned to think of chocolates and desserts as rewards in our childhood. Besides the endorphins released from eating the sweet tasting desserts, the remembered emotional comfort and warmth we received when a caring parent intervened, offering us desserts doubles the amount of the endorphin release.

Sometimes we feel guilty, weak, and disappointed with ourselves when we are trying to lose weight, and start craving for and surrender to the desire to eat sweets. These negative feelings tend to rob us of the pleasure we could have received from eating, and eating itself becomes the cause of more anxiety and tension.

Generally, people do what they know and what they have trained themselves to do. Many people have developed the habit of eating sweets as a main source of their endorphin supply to counteract their pain. Some people develop the habit of taking a walk when encountering negative feelings. There are others who use alcohol, tobacco, and other drugs to counteract their pain. Many others resort to prayer, meditation, or solitude. Others perhaps talk to a brother, sister, a friend, a Rabbi, a Priest, or a therapist. We stand to gain the most benefits when we learn to *constructively* deal with our pain.

Many people become accustomed to leading a reactionary life. They do things in reaction to stressful situations. They become so absorbed in their work and what they must do to keep up with their image of themselves, that they forget how to relate and reap joy from their everyday life. As adults we often expect too much from ourselves, we often "bite off more than we can chew", which often becomes the cause of our disappointments and negative feelings. Then we resort to a quick fix of endorphins from the easiest source we can find. We eventually reach a point at which any action we are about to do that requires effort is considered a negative and a stressful act. We automatically pull out a cigarette when faced with a task. To face the day we drink coffee, take a couple of drinks before a business meeting, and no longer do things just for the fun of it. We start to form reactive habits as a measure to release the pressures that build up from having to deal with day to day tasks. Many people have lost their abilities to generate fun for the sake of having fun. The happiness that they experienced as children from running, jumping, and racing the wind are forgotten.

Many philosophers and behavior experts often tell us that we need to capture the child within us in order to be happy. What they are telling us is that we should, like children, do things for the fun of it. We should aim to capture the fun aspect of everything we do. *We should do things for the sake of enjoying them and learning from them.* When indulging in habits to counteract our negative feelings, we become emotionally weak and seek temporary relief by an artificially induced endorphin rush.

When we depend on our habits to supply us with the endorphins that we need to elevate our mood and emotions, we are no longer in a position to plan and avoid conflicts but to rather subjectively cope with our problems. We need to do things so we can receive pleasure, feel happy and fulfilled on a continuous basis. We need to stop *reacting* to situations in our lives and to start *actively seeking pleasures* which will strengthen our emotional state so we can objectively cope with our day to day pressures. We need to stop *reacting* to situations that we might face in our day to day tasks and become *active* in our pleasure-seeking endeavours.

Overcoming Our Negative Feelings

The most rewarding solutions to problems come about from dealing with conflicts in an objective manner. To be objective, we need to rise above the conflict. We need to have a balanced frame of mind, a calm attitude, and a constructive approach.

We cannot deal with conflicts in our lives when we are feeling emotionally down, or cling to old habits to solve our problems. It is essential that we prepare ourselves to deal with all of life's little problems *constructively.* We can easily fortify our emotional well-being by living our lives fully and by enjoying our experiences.

We need to learn to "stop and smell the roses". Our day to day lives are full of treasured moments that we neglect and forsake. We need to take time and realize these moments that give us joy and happiness. Barbara De Angelis (1994) in her book "Real Moments" describes how to capture our important moments by being present physically and mentally during all the acts that we do. We need to stop being so preoccupied in our day to day living, always ahead of ourselves, planning our next task while still doing the present one. By focusing on what we do, and being present in body and mind to cherish and enjoy our relationships and interactions with our loved ones, we can seize our moments of happiness and joy.

We also need to take a periodic stock of our lives and set our priorities straight. We should examine circumstances that caused us to experience negative feelings, and constructively plan to avoid placing ourselves in such situations again. Very often, just by knowing that we can prevent a conflict from ever happening to us again, we take heart and feel positive. We should also choose to become optimists and develop a habit of dwelling on the positive aspects in our lives rather than the negatives.

A planned calendar full of fun activities can provide us with enough endorphins to set a positive mood and feel good about ourselves. It is essential that we plan our lives and give ourselves time to enjoy our experiences and fortify ourselves with pleasant feelings, so that we can be ready to tackle unpleasantness effectively.

Even when we might not feel up to doing anything,

if we just push ourselves to make a little effort to get out of our gloomy feelings, we soon will start enjoying ourselves. We could start perhaps with a little exercise or any activity that we might enjoy. Once we start to feel the endorphin rush we will start to thoroughly enjoy what we are doing. In order to reach the point where we start enjoying ourselves, we should not give up quickly, we need to indulge ourselves a little in whatever we are doing. Forget about all of life's encumbrances that we have to tackle, and do not worry what other people might think of you. Focus on whatever you are doing and stay with it. When you focus on reaping fun and enjoyment from your activities, you will soon realize that you have become absorbed in what you are doing and begin to thoroughly enjoy yourself. You will realize that you can find joy in the simple things like walking, hiking, swimming, dancing, painting, listening to music or to your friends, sharing their experiences and growing.

Yes growing! Our nerve endings and dendrites are branching out and growing. The belief that our brain cells stop growing as we grow older is not true. Scientists are discovering that the body rule, "use it or lose it," applies to brain cells as well. When certain brain cells are damaged by disease or accident, neighboring brain cells grow and compensate, allowing the accident or stroke victims to regain considerable control of the functions that were lost as a result of damage to the nerve and brain cells. Our activities will stimulate our senses and the electrochemical currents traveling through our nerve pathways will manufacture the happiness causing neurochemicals that elevate our moods and give us a positive outlook. We can then relate to ourselves and others around us in a more positive way. We will strengthen our relationship with the people around us and our attitudes toward our everyday activities. Our daily tasks will no longer be regarded as chores, but rather as sources of pleasure. We will look forward to doing them. We will soon be ready to get out of our reactive habits and give up smoking, drinking coffee or alcohol, and eating in order to feel better.

Easier said than done. It can be very difficult to change a reactive habit, which has likely become an automatic reaction, that supplies us with the momentarily needed endorphins to counteract our pain. When we approach each reactive habit in a well-fortified state of mind, with a good supply of endorphins obtained from the various activities that we enjoy, we will be able to take control of our lives, and tackle any negative feelings that we might have to face, instead of merely coping with our downfalls.

Changing our habits and lifestyle does not happen overnight. To find pleasure, we need to accomplish two things which must be addressed simultaneously because one strengthens the other. One is to confront our negative thoughts and unresolved conflicts so we can relate to ourselves and others in a positive, warm, loving, and cheerful manner. Secondly, we should train ourselves to be present, body, mind, and soul in whatever we are doing so we are present to reap the rewards, the joy and bonding with our loved ones. We need to take time to enjoy our accomplishments.

We also must take time to reflect on our problems and negative feelings in order to resolve them and not to dwell on them, feeling sorry for ourselves and wallowing in our own misery. When reflecting on what causes us pain and suffering, we must rationalize and understand our feelings and conflicts in order to rid ourselves of their burdens. Realize that you have the strength to overcome suffering and can objectively and constructively deal with your problems from the past and the present to become the wiser from them.

It was mentioned in Chapter 1 that muscles use energy in two ways. Internal work includes the maintenance of muscle tone and posture, shivering, and other vegetative processes like digestion and circulation. External work includes moving the body voluntarily and changing body position in the external world. We have also stated that we do not have control over the internal work. However, we do have indirect control. We can influence our muscles and posture, by the way we conduct our thoughts and handle personal conflicts. Sometimes we can become so involved with emotional problems and release neurochemicals which will make us tense and keyed up. Tremendous energy can be used by our muscles when we are tense and keyed up. Such tensions will deplete blood glucose, which often leads to short tempers and frustration. It is during our trying moments that we resort to quick-fix endorphin releasing habits such as smoking or snacking on sweets. Many overweight people have gained large amounts of their weight during times when they were facing difficulties in their lives.

Chapter 18

Stop Being Reactive and Become Active

We can effectively ease tension that is caused by unpleasant thoughts by consciously concentrating on pleasant thoughts. My wise mother used to say "Imagine that you have a shoulder bag with one pouch in the front and another pouch in the back. Place all the pleasant things in your life in the front pouch, so you may pull them out and reminisce and remember them often. Place all the unhappy thoughts and all the things that cause you grief in the back pouch. Heavy loads are better carried on our backs. If you keep your grudges in front, you will trip and fall. And remember my child," she would say, "don't be so hard on yourself, stop every now and then and unload yourself."

We must learn to recognize when we are becoming tense, worried, and keyed up. We need to know what makes us angry and frustrated and learn to deal with these situations *rationally and constructively*. It is not enough to tell someone not to worry, because they cannot just stop worrying. But planning to have a pleasurable adventure on our agenda, we will not find time to worry. By leading a full and more meaningful life, we will allow ourselves to continuously release the endorphins that we need to lift up our moods, and be ready and able to rise above problems and solve them more constructively.

One way we can ensure that we will always have the endorphins that help us cope with trying circumstances in our lives, is to ensure that the brain has the nutrients required to manufacture those endorphins which maintain our positive mood and mental well-being. Therefore, it is essential that we maintain constant supplies of energy for the brain. We can do this in four ways:

1. Eating whole grain foods will ensure a steady supply of slow release glucose into the bloodstream without triggering the release of insulin (see chapter 19 Whole Grain Carbohydrate Source).

2. Choosing activities that require physical exercise will benefit us in three ways:

   (a) It will develop the muscles to increase their mitochondria so that muscles can burn fat more readily.

   (b) It improves the cardiovascular system, supplying the muscles with all the oxygen required to continue relying on a fat energy source, leaving the blood sugar exclusively for the brain's use.

   (c) The exercise itself causes the body to produce endorphins.

3. Consciously planning to break the habit of reactive behavior by replacing it with activities which can generate equivalent amounts of pleasure.

4. Making a conscious effort to dwell on the positive aspects of our lives and remembering our blessings, instead of dwelling on our downfalls and becoming tense and keyed up.

We can start to change our reactionary habits and replace them with activities that are rewarding. No matter how much we try to act positively in our lives and attempt to forget incidents that caused us grief, we cannot totally escape the conditioned behaviors that are routinely built into the brain to respond to the stress of pain, anxiety, and excitement. Food and other quick fixes reward us with the calming effect of opiates that soothe our pain and reduce excitement. By consciously developing the habit of going for a walk or doing some sort of physical exercise, we provide the momentary endorphins usually released from the reactionary habits that we have developed. Slochower and Kaplan, (1980) advise that if those who eat under stress can identify and give a name to the condition that triggers their eating during stressful conditions, they will feel that they have some control over their habit, and are not as likely to overeat.

Try resorting to comedy and making light of tense situations. A momentary relief from stress by diversion, can often decimate tension and ease the severity of a stressful situation.

Chapter 19

Effects Of Sugar On Our Diet

Refined Sugar

Our body mechanisms do not know how to metabolize refined sugar in the quantities we are
consuming today. Only during the past four to five hundred years, has refined sugar become an integral part
of the human diet. The evolutionary development of
man's metabolic systems has been going on for millions
years. Before we began to consume large quantities of
refined sugar, human beings received their glucose
needs from the complex carbohydrates found in grains,
vegetables, and seeds. The only sugars consumed were
found in fruits and honey. During our evolutionary development there was no advantage to having developed mechanisms to deal with eating large quantities
of refined sugars.

Sugar is believed to have been first manufactured
in India in 3000 BC from sugar cane. A Greek General, Nearchus, who traveled to India with Alexander
the Great around 400 BC, tells of "a reed that produces honey without the aid of bees." Sugar was also
developed independently from sugar cane in the Solo-
mon Islands in the South Pacific. A local legend there
suggests that the human race was generated from a

sugar cane stalk. One bud grew and became man. Sugar making spread from India to Indo-China and then Arabia. During the 8th Century the Arabs introduced sugar cane to Spain and southern France, and sugar making spread from there to the rest of Europe. Venice became the center for sugar refining in Europe. The whole world eventually got on the sucrose bandwagon.

In 1493, Christopher Columbus, during his second voyage, brought sugar cane to the New World. In 1544, a sugar refinery was established in London, England, and in 1689, another sugar refinery was established in New York.

Refining sugar played a powerful role in making or breaking economic powers. The establishment of sugar refineries in the West Indies and Southern United States fuelled the slave trade. People from Africa were brought to the New World to work in the sugar plantations and cotton fields that were spreading in the Islands of the West Indies and parts of the United States, wherever there was a warm, moist climate to grow sugar cane. The might of nations and their economic wealth, and the misery of the slaves, was built on refining and trading sugar. Today sugar is produced in many countries throughout the world.

Table sugar is a sweet tasting crystalline whose chemical formula is $C_{21}H_{22}O_{11}$. Table sugar is a disaccharide, composed of a glucose molecule and fructose. Sucrose naturally appears in many fruits and vegetables, and some grains. Sugar is now manufactured in large quantities and comes in many forms and various grades and shades. Golden colored liquid sugar is manufactured for domestic use as refinery syrup. More than 2,000,000 tones of liquid sugar are manufactured in the U.S. annually to be used in ready-made commercial foods. Japan produces 1,000,000 tones of fine grain white sugar annually. The industrial liquid form of sugar is used in all kinds of foods and carbonated beverages and the manufacturing of wine, liquors, and candies, and is added to many desserts that we buy ready-made or prepare at home, such as cakes, cookies, desserts, chocolate bars, and juices. It is widely used in masking the taste of children's medications, especially in cough syrups. Sugar is added to bread, tomato ketchup, and salad dressing. Almost every recipe contains sugar to sweeten the taste of foods. We sprinkle sugar over breakfast cereal and on fruit. Newborn babies are often introduced to sugar water before they are introduced to their mothers' breast milk. Although the use of refined sugar is commonplace to us now, on an evolutionary timescale it is only recently that human beings have developed a taste for sweets.

Prior to refined sugar, the diets of humans included sweet tastes found only in fruits and honey, which contain glucose molecules. Human body mechanisms developed to process glucose only in moderate amounts. During millions of years of evolutionary history, our blood glucose was driven from eating carbohydrates found in grains and seeds, and from lactose and fructose found in milk and fruits. The consumption of refined sugar with almost everything we eat is comparatively new. Our metabolism is ill-equipped to metabolize sugar in the quantities we eat it today.

Chapter 19

Our Bodies Are Very Sensitive To Glucose

We have evolved with mechanisms that closely monitor glucose levels in our blood. As was mentioned in Chapter 7, diabetics suffer from the inability to control their blood sugar, and their blood glucose often rises to unacceptable levels. The long term effects of high blood sugar are dangerous and cause many circulatory, vascular, and kidney complications with devastating consequences. High blood sugar will adversely effect the cells of our bodies because it increases the density of the blood, causing extracellular fluids to disperse into the blood vessels through osmosis, thereby dehydrating our body cells. Also, when blood sugar levels rise above normal, glucose starts to spill over into the urine from the kidneys. Sugar in the urine is the hallmark of people suffering from diabetes. Glucose in the urine exerts osmotic effects and draws more water from the blood into the urine. This markedly reduces the blood volume and further condenses the blood in the blood vessels leading to severe dehydration. Dehydration of cells causes degenerative vascular lesions in the body affecting primarily the fine linings of the retina of the eye, leading to blindness, damaging the fine filtration mechanisms in the kidneys causing high blood pressure and even premature death. When the fine lining of blood vessels are scarred, fat molecules can then lodge in these scars and reduce the circumference of the blood vessels even further, causing circulatory problems, stroke, and coronary artery disease. In extreme cases gangrene in the extremities results from poor circulation and dehydration. We tend to blame fat and cholesterol for blocking blood vessels, but high blood sugar levels are just as much to blame for damaging and scarring body cells and vascular tissue. Low blood sugar levels cause irritability and drastically reduced blood sugar leads to coma and death.

Our body mechanisms react very quickly to reduce the high blood sugar level in the circulatory system after a meal. People not suffering from diabetes have mechanisms that trigger the release of insulin as soon as their bodies sense the entry of glucose into their systems. Insulin is released to counteract sugar and remove sugar from the circulation quickly by allowing the body to burn all the sugars consumed from a meal first and then convert what it can into glycogen, storing some in the liver. We can store about three to four hundred calories of glucose in the liver as glycogen and muscles also store glycogen to be used as energy during intense exercise.

Before refined sugar came on the scene, an average person would obtain their carbohydrates by eating a little fruit, and maybe a little honey, and some whole grains, such as seeds, beans, and other slow-release carbohydrates. If the person was a carnivore, some of the proteins would break up to be burned for energy use. The taste buds would encounter only a little sugar in a meal. The bulk of our blood glucose would be driven from slow-release carbohydrate sources.

Our bodies were designed to work like this: as soon as our taste buds taste sweet, our bodies release insulin. In turn, insulin stops our bodies from using fat for energy and switches all body cells to start using glucose until blood glucose levels begin to drop slowly. As the carbohydrates consumed in the whole grain meal are slowly digested, and the starches are converted to glucose, blood sugar is slowly replaced, maintaining a constant blood sugar level without the release of additional insulin.

Our diet has changed. The bulk of our blood glucose is driven from processed carbohydrates and refined sugars. We do not eat enough slow-release carbohydrates. We now eat large quantities of sugar and processed carbohydrates, and very little, if any whole grains in a meal. Besides adding sugar to everything we eat, we constantly drink sweet tasting beverages, chew sweet tasting gums, and keep popping breath fresheners into our mouths in between meals. These actions will result in continuously triggering our insulin release mechanisms. As we know, the release of insulin switches all body cells to burn glucose, thus we do not give ourselves a chance to burn our body fat.

Because our diet does not contain seeds and whole grains that will release their glucose slowly, our blood sugar levels fluctuate from an extreme high when we start to eat, to an extreme low when all the sugar is utilized and there is no further release of glucose into the blood from digesting grains. We feel hungry soon after we eat a meal which is saturated with sugar.

Our body mechanisms are not designed to deal with the consumption of large quantities of sugar and very small quantities of slow-release carbohydrates. The only mechanism we have that deals with large quantities of sugar is the automatic release of large quantities of insulin which lowers blood sugar level drastically. Since our diet is often lacking slow-release carbohydrates, we quickly deplete our blood sugar level and feel hungry soon after we eat. We do not have mechanisms that can store more glycogen to supply energy to our brain on a longer term basis. Nor do we have a mechanism that tells the body "hold down your insulin, there will be a shortage of glucose soon because there were not enough grains and complex carbohydrates consumed with the meal." Therefore, adding sugar to our food poses a major problem. Our body mechanisms are developed to release insulin according to the size of the meals we consume and the taste of sweet that we experience. Eating large amounts of sugar and sweets triggers the release of large amounts of insulin. The continuous eating and tasting sweet, continuously triggers the release of insulin, and prevents our bodies from burning fat.

Whole Grain Carbohydrate Source

We require an uninterrupted supply of glucose to provide our brain cells with energy. The slightest shortage of energy to the brain interferes with the production of endorphins and other neurochemicals. When we develop a taste for whole grain meals, we will automatically seek this very friendly carbohydrate source which ensures a steady, constant supply of energy to the brain, which will lead us to experience a state of calm emotional well-being.

Whole grain foods are any edible grains that are coarsely crushed or ground, but still contain the outer skin. Our bodies are designed to acquire glucose energy mainly from whole grain foods which break down to glucose. Whole grain foods are also a good source of vitamin B complex, and other vitamins. Whole grain foods are very beneficial to our health because the bran, which is the outer skin of the kernel, is a good source of dietary fibre, helping to stimulate and activate the large bowels. However, the major health benefit that whole grains offer is their slow release of energy. It takes about half a day to break down whole grain meals and release their starches. This slow release of carbohydrates means that the starches we consume can be converted to glucose very slowly. The steady, slow release of glucose into the blood will not trigger the release of insulin. This makes whole grains an ideal carbohydrate energy source, almost a total brain fuel. Because insulin release is not triggered by the digestion of whole grains, muscles continue to burn fat, and blood sugar will be used exclusively by the brain.

The fiber hypothesis suggests that unrefined carbohydrate foods protect us against many diseases such as colon cancer and cardiovascular disease. It must also be the steady supply of neurochemicals that protects us from cancer, since neurochemicals also control our immune system.

When eating whole grain foods, the grains must be cracked or crushed and the skins partly removed to expose the complex carbohydrate content. If we eat whole grains without breaking the husks we will not be able to digest them properly before they leave the digestive tract and we will not be able to reap the benefit of their energy.

Breakfast cereals that contain a variety of grains,

such as Robin Hood's Red River Cereal, Rogers' Nine Grain Cereal, are considered total brain foods, since they provide both the proteins and the slow release of glucose necessary for brain activities and the manufacturing of neurochemicals and endorphins. The mix of the grains ensures the presence of all the essential amino acids from which the body can make its own body-protein (see Chapter 2 Protein), and the slow release of carbohydrates enables the body to maintain a constant blood sugar level for a considerable length of time without triggering further release of insulin, providing the brain with all the energy it requires and delaying sensations of hunger. Nebisco's Cream Of Wheat, Oatmeal, and other whole grain cereals taken with milk or protein source also have the same effect.

Preventative medicine clinics have found that their clients were able to lose weight when they were placed on diets containing whole grains. Whole grain foods have been found to be very therapeutic in the treatment of people with mood disorders, hyperactive children, manic depressive individuals, and also people with metabolic disorders and diabetes.

The Desire to Eat Sweets

When we open a box of chocolates, our intention is to eat only one or maybe two chocolates, but as soon as we taste one piece many of us will come back for more until the whole box is eaten. Despite our determination not to eat sweets, once we start eating them we are compelled to eat them and feel disappointed when the box is empty. There are two factors that make us return to the chocolate box for more.

One is the release of endorphins from eating sweets. Just like the rat in Olds' experiment (in Chapter 3), we will repeat the actions that give us pleasure. The other reason we keep eating chocolate is because of its sweet taste. As soon as we eat a piece of chocolate the release of insulin is triggered, our metabolism shifts to burn glucose instead of fat. When the body burns glucose, it quickly depletes blood sugar, and we feel hungry for sweets to raise the blood sugar levels again. The role of insulin in utilizing sugar energy in the body can throw a person into a "catch-22". You eat sugar and you release insulin, insulin in turn lowers the blood sugar, which makes you feel hungry and you crave sugar and so on. As this scenario is going on, the body is unable to burn any fat.

The Taste of Sweet & The Metabolism of Fat

We release insulin every time we experience the taste of sweet, and insulin in turn stops the body from burning fat. Many people underestimate the effects of eating sugar on their metabolism. They often refer to sugar as just "empty calories", because its caloric content is only four calories per gram of sugar and the body burns sugar as soon as it enters the body. Instead they focus their attention on refraining from eating fat. No one argues against the fact that fat has more calories, and whatever we eat in fat becomes directly deposited in our fat cells, and we will only use fat for our energy when the release of insulin is suppressed and all the sugars consumed are used first. Once we accumulate a large quantity of fat, we find it difficult to get rid of it if we keep eating sugar. The taste of sweet is the culprit that prevents us from burning fat.

Of course, by eating less fat we will reduce the amount of fat that will be deposited in the body. But by eating less fat we will not burn the excess fat which has been already accumulated in our fat cells if we keep on eating sugars. When people constantly eat sweets, their muscles will burn glucose. Therefore the answer to allowing our bodies to have a chance to burn fat is to include a slow-release carbohydrate source in each meal, and especially in meals that taste sweet, so that when the effects of insulin subside, slow-release carbohydrates will continue to replenish the blood glucose without the release of more insulin. This way, our bodies will resume burning fat and will reserve blood sugar exclusively for the brain so that we can go for much longer periods of time without feeling hungry.

Giving Ourselves the Advantage

I would like to urge the readers to try it out for themselves and refrain from eating anything that tastes sweet except for some fruit and juices, and include whole grain cereal in your diet for two or three days. You will experience the results first hand. You will feel much more energetic and far less hungry, and experience a calmer, and a more content state of mind.

Although my objective in this book is to emphasize that each person must become responsive to their own body needs by responding to their sensations of hunger and cravings, the taste of sweet is an exception. Humans have been developing a taste for sweet and abusing it on a grand scale for the past few hundred years. We owe it to ourselves to at least develop a taste for the type of foods that our ancestors have been surviving on for millions of years.

We need to give ourselves the advantage of developing a taste for the foods that our bodies are familiar with, foods that our bodies have the mechanisms to best digest, absorb, and utilize. For millions of years the human body was developing mechanisms to deal with grains, seeds, and slow-release carbohydrates. We cannot deny ourselves these foods now simply because we have manufactured and refined table sugar, and have become attracted to the taste of sweet.

Eating sugar is a double whammy: we release neurochemicals *from* eating sweets and *for* eating sweets. Sugar is a brain nutrient: the sole source of brain energy. We also release serotonin, a powerful mood elevating and pain suppressing endorphin, while eating sweets. Therefore we must make a conscious effort to recognize and differentiate between our emotional hunger and nutritive hunger when it comes to the reasons why we eat sweets.

During the past few decades we have changed our diets and we are consuming much more fat, protein, and carbohydrates than our ancestors did. Also most of the carbohydrates that we eat are processed. When we do not eat whole grain, we quickly digest and absorb the carbohydrates eaten and raise our blood sugar triggering the release of insulin, making us feel hungry soon after we eat. The fat in our diet is directly deposited in our fat cells and our bodies do not have a chance to burn it.

Fat is not used by our brain cells and does not interfere directly in the energy processes required to release neurochemicals. We do not become conditioned to eat fat as we do to eating sugar and glucose. We only crave for foods that contain fat every now and then, whenever there is a shortage of fat soluble vitamins in our bodies. We also crave foods which contain proteins when our bodies are short of proteins.

Our craving for sugar is triggered by a drop in blood sugar caused by eating sugar. Eating sugar makes us want to eat more sugar. Our blood sugar levels fluctuate as we eat sweets and our body reacts to eating sweets by lowering our blood sugar levels and subsequently we crave for more sweets, taking us on an emotional roller coaster. We feel high when our blood sugar rises and we feel low as blood sugar levels come down.

Many people think that they are addicted to sugar and they say that they have a sweet tooth. The body does not become addicted to sugar as it can become addicted to drugs. Remember in Chapter 4 (The Reinforcing Mechanisms of the Body), we talked about addiction and how neurons tend to develop tolerance to repeated excitatory stimuli. A person using a drug requires increasingly larger doses of the drug to attain the same feeling of elation. If drug users do not keep increasing the doses of the drug to which they have developed a tolerance, they will experience withdrawal symptoms. Refraining from eating sugar will certainly not cause any withdrawal symptoms, nor will we need to increase our glucose consumption to experience elation. Our body mechanisms regulate blood glucose levels. After we eat certain nutrients we develop a dislike for them until there is a need for those nutrients again. We all have experienced a sort of dislike, even a sick feeling after gorging on chocolates and sweets, but after a while, when our blood sugar starts to fall, we again start to crave sweets.

Our taste for sweets is a learned habit. It is a habit that we like because sweet tasting foods contain glucose, the only fuel source the brain can use. Rewards and punishments are imprinted upon children as a result of having or not having sweets and desserts. If we were good and did what we were told, we were worthy of cake, chocolates, candy, and dessert. Many children were often punished by being denied desserts. If they misbehaved they were denied chocolate, candy and other goodies. When poked by a needle in the doctor's office, a candy sucker was often stuck in a child's mouth, to pacify the hurt and indignity he or she had endured. Children grow up psychologically conditioned to sweet tasting goodies and junk.

The taste for sweet is learned. If we were able to develop a taste for sweets, we should be able to develop a taste for slow-release carbohydrates as well! These foods can have just as powerful an effect on the emotional well-being of a person. Although the results from eating slow-release carbohydrates are not as instantaneous as eating table sugar, the uninterrupted supply of energy to the brain from slow-release carbohydrates is more rewarding.

The Regulation of Blood Sugar Level

Glucose is used by every cell in the body. It provides cells with the fuel necessary to carry out the functions necessary for survival. Our bodies must maintain acceptable levels of blood glucose. If our blood glucose concentrations fall below normal, we will feel hungry. If blood sugar levels rise above normal, we will feel sleepy. If the blood sugar is pushed to the limits of either extreme, we will go into a coma. Hypoglycemia is caused by low blood sugar levels. Hyperglycemia is caused when blood sugar rises above acceptable levels. Optimal functioning is attained when blood sugar remains in an acceptable range between 70 -100 mg per 100 ml.

Our bodies regulate our own blood glucose levels automatically. Diabetics lose the ability to regulate their own blood sugar because their insulin production is affected and they do not produce enough insulin to meet their bodies' needs. Only a person who is suffering from diabetes needs to intervene in the regulation of their blood glucose.

People who are not diabetics could not interfere with their blood sugar levels even if they tried. The regulation of blood sugar is an innate mechanism. Even if we eat large quantities of sugar our blood sugar will rise only for a short time. The insulin triggering mechanisms work very quickly and force the body to burn sugar instead of fat, and also instruct liver cells to convert all excess sugars to glycogen. When blood sugar begins to fall, the hormone glucagon takes over and slowly allows glycogen from the liver to supply and maintain blood sugar levels, and allows our body cells to burn fat for energy. This regulates and maintains blood sugar at an acceptable level.

However, the way we eat and the way we expend our energy, can help our bodies to maintain our blood glucose levels with minimum stress. When we feel hungry we should eat, and when we eat, we should not load ourselves with refined sugars that will cause the release of large quantities of insulin. We should eat carbohydrates that will slowly release their glucose into the blood and maintain steady levels of blood sugar for several hours at a time. We can exercise our muscles so they may reach their maximum potential to store their own glycogen in sufficient quantities, and develop more mitochondria to burn fat more effectively. We must improve the capacity of our hearts and lungs to deliver oxygen and other nutrients to the muscles and remove waste. Muscles will not then draw on the liver glycogen during intense exercise, causing a drop in blood sugar levels. When muscles are burning fat, they leave the blood sugar level alone. A constant supply of energy and nutrients to the brain will allow it do its work, and we will feel content and happy.

Chapter 20

The Diet Industry's Gimmicks

The Diet Industry's Gimmicks

A multibillion dollar diet industry, and to some extent the fashion industry, have been employing the media and targeting us with advertisements designed to convince us to diet and lose weight. The reason many people gain weight is because they believe the gimmicks and false illusions these industries present. They make us believe that in order to look good and be slim we must control our diet and restrict the calories we eat. They are wrong. We do not have to restrict the calories in our diet in order to burn excess body fat and develop attractive figures. By controlling our food intake, we are likely to become susceptible to weight gain and fall prey to the diet industry's money making schemes. Our bodies have an innate intelligence that has been developing for millions of years, designing self-regulatory mechanisms to ensure our health and well-being as a whole. By attempting to control body weight through manipulating food intake, we often interfere and retard many of our innate mechanisms, and cause ourselves more harm.

Most of the diet industry's gimmicks are designed with one thing in mind: to take your money and make you dependent! These people have many gadgets and other ineffective or half effective methods to help you lose weight while constantly "keeping their hands in your pockets." They have many schemes to make you buy their silly goods at super-inflated prices. Their goods sometimes are nothing more than placebos that make you think you are getting something for your money. Often you end up paying dearly for a little bit of ordinary food in a plastic bag, a frozen dinner in a tray, dried dinners in a pouch, a liquid meal in a can. They also charge you for advice, for teaching you how to tolerate hunger-pangs, and how to starve yourself and continue with a self-imposed famine. They train you in self-hypnosis so you can curb your appetite and continue your starvation regimes. They trick you into buying lotions that they claim will melt fat when applied to your skin. There is no end to their schemes. They have a new invention every day to make you part with your hard earned cash. Special gels in capsules are sold which supposedly stick to foods in the stomach to prevent the foods from being digested and absorbed by the body. They sell you foods that swell in your stomach and make you uncomfortable so you cannot eat anything else. There are over-the-counter diet candies that contain a local anesthetic to numb your taste buds so you cannot taste sweets properly. Perhaps this is their best invention yet, although it retards our natural mechanisms which control eating. They also sell electric vibrators to be applied to various parts of the body to shape up and tone wasted muscles. They have invented hot wraps to help remove your cellulite. If only you realize that there is no such thing as cellulite!

When we ignore a craving sensation designed to

lead us to eat according to the body's cellular require-ments, our bodies learn to cope without the nutrients they require by lowering the metabolic rate. As we now know, a lowered metabolic rate renders our bodies sus-ceptible to weight gain, and then we become life-long customers of the diet industry's gimmicks.

Each person has unique and different metabolic and nutritional needs. No two people are alike. No one knows what experiences any other person has had, or how they feel, and what innate nutritional requisitions they have at any given time. How can anyone, other than ourselves, know what we need to eat, when only we know what our innate requisitions are? Dietary needs change according to our experiences. We must realize that we cannot control our weight by following a diet menu prepared for us by others. Our dietary needs are innate requisitions reflected in our cravings and thoughts, and we are the only ones who know how to satisfy these requisitions.

Every day we hear something new about various foods and substances that are thought to be anti-can-cer agents or good for us - the next miracle food. Many specialists that were recommending we eat certain foods because they were antioxidants and prevent cancer or some other disease are now saying the opposite. If there was an anti-cancer agent in our food, our taste buds would probably recognize it by its taste. Our hypotha-lamus, together with our cerebral cortex, will make us crave for it whenever it becomes needed at the cellular level. By responding to all our innate sensory messages, and eating the foods that we crave, we will receive the nourishment our bodies require, including substances that help the body to build its immune system and fight cancer.

Our Bodies Can Defend Themselves

We might think of ourselves as fragile human beings unable to survive on our own in a harsh environment. We might think that we need to seek the help of others to become healthy and fit. We are not as fragile as we think. On the contrary, our bodies have systems with capabilities beyond belief, designed to protect and guard us from illnesses and disease. Our immune system, as we have been discovering lately, is equipped and able to defend us from illness and diseases with mechanisms of incomprehensible sophistication and precision. All our body mechanisms are interdependent. Our immune system is totally dependent on our innate mechanisms that control our eating. The immune system would be powerless and useless without an equally sophisticated and precise mechanism of supply and services, providing all the nutrients necessary to help fight off disease and infections.

Our bodies are designed with all the mechanisms necessary to ensure our health and well-being. We have first class detecting and sensory mechanisms which examine and monitor our internal and external environment. We even monitor the air we breathe. Our noses are so sensitive we can smell garlic odor at concentrations of one molecule in 50,000 million. We can detect more than ten thousand different odors. We monitor the foods we eat with our ten thousand taste buds situated at the gate of our food intake, inspecting every speck of food that we eat or drink. Our taste buds are equipped to distinguish all the different foods that we eat by sensing and differentiating the molecular structures of foods. We have many sensory detectors spread throughout our bodies, monitoring and informing us of the various needs that we have. We have mechanisms that regulate our nutritional intake by triggering sensations of specific hunger and satiation. Our sensory organs constantly monitor temperature, light, sound, touch, blood glucose levels, and all other homeostatic conditions, and innately trigger hormones and neurochemicals to maintain homeostatic conditions, ensuring our health and well-being. We monitor our environment, keep a record of our findings, and formulate a plan of defense and adaptation according to the conditions we experience. Our reaction to our environment includes immediate action and preparation for future action when we encounter the same conditions again. In other words, *we are capable of innately learning and using what we have experienced to take care of ourselves.*

Our immune system, for example, is capable of actual combat. When a foreign bacteria or protein that can cause us harm enters our internal space, our immune system prepares for war. A scout team sneaks up on the invader and tags it with a chemical. The body then manufactures antibodies tailored specifically to attack the intruder. Our immune system triggers the release of special white blood cells called T-cells, which arise from the thymus gland and regulate our whole immune system. Killer T-cells are released and directly attach themselves to foreign or abnormal cells. These killer T-cells confront the intruding enemy cells just

like kamikazes on a suicide mission. They attach themselves to the intruding enemy cells, killing themselves
and the enemy with them. There is also a third group
of T-cells, called the helper T-cells, which supervise
the warfare and control the formation of antibodies.
Helper T-cells go all about our bodies stimulating our
body cells to produce B-cells. B-cells keep shooting out
sticky substances that bind and capture prisoners by
grouping the enemy cells together. Other big white cells
are also released from the bone marrow. These scaven-
gers eat the debris and clean up after the war when the
battle is won. Our defense mechanisms are as interesting and as advanced, if not more so, than the sophisticated Star Wars, Smart Weapons, and missiles that we
have witnessed in Operation Desert Storm during the
Gulf War. Our bodies not only fight our wars, they keep
records of our strategies and automatically use these
strategies in future to defend ourselves.

The mechanisms that control our food intake are
just as sophisticated as the mechanisms that control
our immune system. They work in concert with each
other. For example, when we catch a cold or develop
an infection, we do not feel like eating. All our energy
becomes directed towards building antibodies and preparing our immune system to fight off the infection.
After a little while we develop specific cravings and a
desire to eat specific foods. Some people might crave
for pineapple juice, others look for orange juice, boiled
eggs, perhaps some chicken, parsley, mint, or passion
fruit depending on what their bodies have learned to
eat in the past to replenish the nutrients used to fight
off infection. We see this type of behavior in animals

and house pets. For example a dog might refrain from eating for a little while when feeling sick, then start to eat grass in order to get well.

Our digestive system, together with many other sensory mechanisms, including smell, taste, and the various monitoring centers throughout the body, become very sensitive during an illness. Certain tastes and smells become either desirable or intolerable. We might feel a quiver in our stomach if we attempt to eat anything that is undesirable.

When we are not using our first class equipment designed to regulate our dietary and other mechanisms essential to our survival, we lose our abilities of innately knowing what we need to eat and do in order to stay healthy and fit. Remember the body's rule, "Use it or lose it"? Any mechanism, muscle, or tissue not used will atrophy. Once the body has lost the innate ability to fend off illness on its own, we become sick, and must seek appropriate medical intervention. Although the body comes equipped with its own mechanisms for dealing with illness, it does not mean that we do not need medical intervention to help us fight illnesses.

Since the advent of antibiotics and other medications, death from diseases such as pneumonia, and other infections is preventable in many instances. However the medical profession is very much aware that these antibiotics must be administered very cautiously because of the resistance many germs will develop, rendering antibiotics useless. Also, using antibiotics to fight off infection interferes with the development of the body's own natural immunity.

Our food intake mechanisms are well equipped to recognize what nutrients we need to eat, when, and how much. We have the mechanisms that are able to trigger our hunger and specific cravings to meet these requisitions. Why should we not develop our innate abilities to select and choose the required nourishment? It is foolish to resort to haphazard diet regimes and unnatural methods in an ill-fated attempt to regulate our weight and improve our health. Why should we? We already possess the finest class of mechanisms which effectively control our health and well-being.

The good news is, once we relinquish control over our innate physiological mechanisms that control eating, we quickly regain our innate eating skills. We can re-learn to respond innately to our body needs. Once we start to respond to our sensations of craving, and satiation, the endorphins in our bodies increase and we become happier and enjoy our lives more. Once we become happier and more content we become more responsive to our innate requests. When we begin to recognize our own needs more accurately, we will be able to choose with more precision the nutrients our bodies need. We will become more energetic, grow emotionally, and expand our intellectual and social horizons. We will start enjoying our lives instead of constantly torturing ourselves. When we learn to take our eating cues from our physical feelings, we will eat healthy meals and still eat what we want to eat. We will stop looking for something that is going to make us feel better momentarily. We will stop raiding the refrigerator, or run to the doughnut store to boost our system with the much needed endorphins that make us feel happy. We will enjoy physical activities and exercise. We will find a new joy in eating without counting calories and still become healthy, happy, and fit.

Chapter 21

Innate Eating Practices

Respond To Innate Eating Mechanisms

To be responsive to our bodies' innate mechanisms which control eating, means to learn innately what to eat, when to eat, and how much. This pattern of eating is not alien to us. We are designed to seek our nourishment by responding to innate cues which come to mind in the form of hunger, craving, and satiation.

Of course, this does not mean that we should go out and eat everything that we see or think about. We have to aim to become responsive to our sensations of hunger and satiation. We need to develop selective eating skills by recognizing specific cravings. We have been abusing our natural mechanisms that innately control our eating by being insensitive to our own hunger and cravings. In many instances, we have become accustomed to using food to pacify our emotional feelings. Many of us have become academic eaters, and forgotten how to respond to our feelings of hunger. We have become accustomed to eating based upon our knowledge of food in terms of its caloric value, carbohydrate, fat, and protein content, and we have forgotten about the pleasure we receive by eating. We have been eating what we think we should eat and how much we think we should eat, instead of eating what we *feel* we should eat.

We have cluttered our innate recognition of various tastes by attaching caloric and other values to what we eat. We have learned to describe some foods as sinful, and refer to other foods as taboo. We often rate our foods according to the economic and cultural prejudices that we have. Sometimes we eat foods we do not like simply because we are told that they are good for us. We have taught ourselves to relate to food in a different way than our bodies do.

Our bodies recognize and sense food by its taste, smell, color, texture, and the way in which it satisfies our hunger. Also, we have the mechanisms that convey to us our nutritional needs at the cellular level with specific sensations of hunger, craving, and satiation. When we crave for foods, sometimes we can taste the foods we crave for, we can visualize the color, texture, and smell. To respond to our innate mechanisms which control eating, we need to learn to relate to our food in the same manner that our bodies do. We must do away with all the nonessential values that we have learned to attach to food. We must untangle our physical sensations of hunger from our emotional reasons for eating. We need to stop the feelings of guilt that often accompany eating something that we have craved for. We need to allow ourselves to relate to our food in terms of our enjoyment and contentment. *We must eat our food because we like it and not because it is good for us.* As we begin to become responsive to our sensors, our natural abilities will surface and we will be able to select what our bodies require to become healthy.

The Difference Between Academic and Innate Eating

Academic eaters eat only what their calorie counters tell them to eat, often leaving the dinner table unsatisfied. They are unsatisfied because they have not eaten the foods for which their bodies hungered. Their bodies have not received the momentary nutrients they are calling for, even though they may have eaten a variety of nutrients. In fact, they may have eaten everything their bodies could possibly need, and if they happened to be lucky they might have eaten the nutrients that are momentarily required in their bodies. Even then, they might not have eaten sufficient quantities of the required food to satisfy their hunger because they are only allowed limited quantities on their diet menu. Academic eaters remain in a constant battle to refrain from eating. They do not receive satisfaction and pleasure from eating as innate eaters do.

Academic eaters eat because they think it is time to eat. They do not eat because they feel hungry. When people eat when they are not hungry, they cannot be responding to their internal cues and innate sensations of hunger. Nor could they be eating according to their bodies' momentary needs. They will not know if they have had enough to eat because they were not hungry when they started their meal.

On the other hand, when we eat because we feel hungry, we give ourselves the opportunity to reflect on what we want to eat. Thoughts and images of various foods and their tastes pop into our minds, and we feel a desire to eat these foods. These thoughts and images of foods are part of the innate eating cues and sensations, that are triggered by specific shortages of nutrients at the cellular level. When we eat what we want to eat we feel much happier and more satisfied than when we eat foods planned for us in a diet book.

Academic eaters review the caloric values of their food and calculate its carbohydrate, fat, and protein content. They flip the pages in food guides and diet books to find out what they must eat and what they must not. They learn brainwashing techniques so they can control themselves and resist eating what they want to eat, eating only what is specified for them in a special menu.

Innate eaters rely on their imaginations and wake up their cravings to the various foods that might tickle their fancy. They visualize and imagine the tastes of the foods they want to eat. They learn to relate to the taste, texture, and smell of the foods they eat and how their hunger is satisfied. They develop a skill by which they can sense the foods that are momentarily needed in their bodies.

Innate eaters use their built-in sensory network of ten thousand tastebuds, neuronally linked to the hypothalamus and the cortex of the brain. Their innate mechanisms which control eating receive and process all food-related information from the various sensory organs sensing taste, texture, color, and smell, and store all the information in their memory banks. Our hypothalamus also facilitates all food-related information about requisitions and nutrients needed by our various systems and has the mechanisms that will trigger sensations of hunger and satiation, and we can select from the stored data in the brain about foods we have eaten before. Why should we not respond to our innate eating requests? Who knows better than ourselves what nutrients our bodies need?

When we respond to our sensations of hunger and develop our skill of cueing into our innate requisitions, we can choose the foods required by the body - no more, no less. We will be aware of the foods that will satisfy our hunger. We will develop the skill to innately recognize the foods required in our bodies at the cellular level. We will also know that we have delivered to ourselves the nutrients needed by our body cells because the taste and the smell of the foods we eat will feel extra delicious and appetizing, and we will thoroughly enjoy our food, feeling nourished, content, and happy.

When people do not receive the nutrients their bodies need, their hunger persists, and eventually they give in and give up dieting for a while. In starting to eat to replenish their depleted nutritional stores, they often attack food and start to eat everything they find, gorging themselves as if they have a "bottomless pit" within them that cannot be filled. Perhaps they have too many requisitions for various nutrients to fill, and start gobbling everything in sight to meet the demands of their bodies. After gorging themselves, they feel guilty and they punish themselves for eating and begin to starve themselves more. Surely this type of behavior has a negative impact on their physical and psychological well-being.

Many theories have been suggested as to the cause of obesity, including unhappiness and depression. Rodin, Schank, and Striegel-Moore (1989) support the idea that *in overweight people, unhappiness and depression seem to be the result of obesity and not its cause, and dieting behavior only makes problems worse.*

When people subject themselves to inconsistent meal sizes and periodically gorge themselves, they disrupt their insulin production mechanisms. We release insulin at the start of a meal according to the size of the meal we usually eat. Periodic gorging therefore trains our bodies to release large quantities of insulin, often resulting in releasing too much insulin for the size of the meal consumed. As we know, depleting our blood sugar level will lead to craving for sweets shortly after we eat. If we do not replenish the glucose (which you remember is the main source of energy for the brain), we can experience mood swings and periods of frustration and depression. Leaving the brain without proper energy also leads to a lowered metabolic rate. If this is habitually practised through dieting, it renders us to become susceptible to weight gain and we might even become fatter than before we started dieting.

Innate eaters are constantly responding to their inner feelings of hunger, and satiation, they do not experience compulsive eating attacks. Their bodies become accustomed to releasing consistent amounts of insulin according to consistent meal sizes. Therefore, they maintain constant blood sugar levels, avoiding the drastic mood swings which many compulsive eaters experience. Innate eaters therefore remain in a good mood and feel good about themselves. They are calmer, more content, and lead happier lives.

Innate eating mechanisms employ the processes of learning. Innate eaters have learned to cue into the various sensations of hunger and craving, and satiation. They are able to produce more endorphins while eating, and they can receive more enjoyment during eating. (Refer to Chapter 3, Endorphins that Control Eating and Learning Behaviors.)

How Do We Become Innate Eaters?

Innate eating is natural to us, our bodies are designed so that we will recognize our needs through our feelings. When we relinquish conscious control over eating and begin to relate to the more subtle, profound, and complex sensory nature of our bodies, we will start to respond to the mastery of our bodies' design which will guide us to do what we must do to keep happy, healthy, and fit.

Our physiological mechanisms are far too complex and more far reaching than the simplistic knowledge we have about balancing our energy intake to our energy output, and the limited understanding we have about our life-sustaining mechanisms which govern our health and well-being. *Controlling our innate body mechanisms with our limited academic knowledge and understanding cannot do us any good and will only hinder and disrupt our natural abilities,* preventing us from reaching our full potential.

Chapter 21

Removing the self-imposed constraints which limit our potential is easy and attainable: all we have do is to start relating to ourselves through how we feel. When we stop thinking of food in terms of calories, we will automatically relate to food in terms of its taste, texture, smell, and post-ingestional conditioning. When we start relating to food as the substance that nourishes our bodies, we will stop thinking of food in terms of its molecular structure. Instead of becoming concerned about how much food we need to eat, we will start to respond to the way the food is satisfying our hunger. Instead of spending our time calculating and analyzing our meals, we will take time to reflect on the pleasures we receive from eating. Instead of eating foods that we are told are good for us, we will seek out the foods that give us energy and make us feel satisfied. We will avoid foods that can cause allergic reactions or foods we cannot tolerate well. *Innate eating is part of our nature that will surface when we start to respond to sensations of hunger, and satiation.* We might have to re-learn how to relate to our feelings and sensations. But once we get the hang of it, it will become natural for us to effectively respond to our innate sensations and eat the nutrients our bodies need and no more.

Eating is a completely sensuous experience from which we receive great pleasure. It is important that we take time to enjoy this pleasure. Very often we forsake the pleasures of eating by not paying attention to what we eat. We often eat while we are thinking or preoccupied with other things. Many people eat while watching television, paying more attention to the show than to the food they are eating.

Eating is one of the most important and pleasurable experiences in our lives and we take it for granted. Health and nutrition experts keep telling us what foods are good for us and what we must eat. Food connoisseurs give us advice on food presentation and etiquette and how to eat our food. They tell us where to place our cutlery and our wine goblets. These all add to the ambience and enjoyment of eating, however, *the most important aspect of eating, that which gives us the greatest reward, is the very personal experience of how we enjoy our meal.*

The enjoyment we receive from eating has a major role in developing our innate knowledge about the foods we eat. When we eat, we experience sheer joy orchestrated by a symphony of our senses - the satisfaction of our taste buds, the tantalizing of our organs of smell, the mesmerizing sensation of touch, feeling the temperature and texture of the food we are eating. Delight your senses with the sizzle and smell of the barbecue, the crunch of the apple or the pleasurable feel of eating juicy fruits and vegetables. Feast your eyes on the colors of your foods, and relax and enjoy the way your meal satisfies your hunger.

In effect, while we are eating, our taste buds, together with the rest of our sensory mechanisms are compiling an innate vocabulary to facilitate and embed in our memory how to match specific hunger with specific foods and meet the momentary requirements of our bodies, and store the information so we may know what to crave when we need these nutrients again. As we experience craving sensations later on, we can then reflect on our sensations of hunger and cue in to what foods we want and need to eat. Developing our mechanisms which control eating involves innately learning about the foods we eat and recalling these foods later when our bodies require their nutrients.

We cannot effectively undertake to control our eating at will and according to our academic knowledge, since our body metabolism is a totally innate function and our nutritional requirements vary from day to day. This is one of the reasons academic eaters binge every now and then when their bodies can no longer tolerate a self-imposed famine.

We have all the mechanisms to innately learn about the foods we need to eat. Through our feelings of hunger and craving, we sense, recognize, and recall these foods. As we satisfy our needs we experience pleasure. This is the design of our bodies. The pleasure we experience while eating is the most powerful tool we have to positively relate to and learn about the foods we eat. The innate knowledge that we acquire about the foods we eat is the most integral part of a healthy eating behavior that we should strive to strengthen and develop. We have been academically learning about the quality and nutritional value of foods, and ignoring the fact that nutrition also includes the reaction of our bodies to food. *This includes how we are enjoying our food, and how satisfied we feel by eating it.*

When we sit down to eat we must leave our troubles behind, relax, savor and enjoy the food we are eating! We should not think about work or things we have to do, but rather live the moment we are eating, and experience the joy. Once we forget about the caloric or nutritional content of food, we will be amazed at how quickly we start to relate to foods the way our bodies were intended to. We will experience a true pleasure when eating to enjoy rather than being concerned about caloric content.

One morning after breakfast I was sitting quietly in the kitchen, planning my workday and feeling satisfied, content, and cheerful. For some reason I thought of what I had eaten for breakfast and began to add up the calories that I had eaten for breakfast, which did not add up to more than 160. I was comparing my old ways of controlling my weight by calorie counting with the new discovery of eating according to how I felt. Although I was feeling content, full and satiated at that moment, the thought of having only 160 calories struck me as not enough. I should eat more, I thought. The recommended breakfast is about 250 calories. Suddenly I realized that my calm, relaxed, and joyful frame of mind was gradually slipping away as I thought about the calories and the protein content of my meal. I had to quickly stop myself from calculating my meal and begin to focus on how I felt. Relating to my food in terms of calories and proteins was alienating me from a pleasurable, satiated feeling that I was enjoying. I did not like the idea of not being in touch with myself and my feelings. Calorie counting had been robbing me of the joy of experiencing the pleasurable satiated feelings that I now experience after my meals.

Counting calories to control weight is unnatural and strenuous. Hunger means that our bodies require nutrients. It means that we should attend to our needs and start to investigate what to eat, and eat only until we feel satiated.

Chapter 21

When we feel hungry, instead of eating whatever is there to eat, we should practice taking a few moments to relax and reflect upon our feelings of hunger; to examine our feelings.

This might seem odd at first, because we really do not know how to reflect upon our hunger. When you relax you should reflect on how you are feeling, whether you feel hungry, thirsty, or just tired.

About one and a half hours before a meal, many people often stop for a moment and a quick thought crosses their mind that it will soon be time to eat, and they often gauge their work schedule so that they can take a break for lunch or supper. Our body prepares digestive juices and hormones according to the nutritional requirements at the cellular level about one and half hours ahead of a meal time. This means that your body is preparing digestive juices and hormones to receive the next meal (for more details on this process, refer to Chapter 14, Biological Rhythms). Reflecting on what we feel we want to eat when our bodies are preparing our digestive system to receive our next meal allows us to cue in to the nutrients that are needed at the cellular level. Reflect on what you wish to eat. What type of foods would feel nice to eat? Reflect on the taste and the texture of the food you would like to experience, whether you would like something sweet, sour, salty, creamy, crunchy, hot or cold. Think about various tastes that are most desirable at that moment. It is amazing how easily we can choose the exact nutrients required in our body at that moment. We will know first hand that what we have chosen to eat is what we need - our food will taste delicious.

You simply choose what you want to eat from the various foods that come to your mind. If you do not have the food that you feel you want on hand, you could perhaps make a note of it on your shopping list, and think of an alternate food. You have often practised this type of exercise when you eat out at a restaurant. As we question ourselves about how we feel and what we want to eat, we start to learn to automatically choose the foods that are rich in what our bodies need at the cellular level. A flash of a specific food item will come to mind, perhaps a food we have not eaten for a while. As we learn to eat these foods, we will begin to realize that our eating habits are changing. We will start enjoying our meals more, and begin to feel more energetic. As we move away from academic eating practices and start to respond to our cravings and eat what we feel we want to eat, all sorts of foods and tastes will pop into our heads. We may go on a binge for a certain food for perhaps ten days or so, just as the children in Dr. Davis' study (Chapter 1).

Our eating habits change as we continue practising taking our cues from within ourselves. We gradually learn how to work with our own bodies and take care of all our needs. The psychological ramifications of deciding what you want to eat instead of refraining from eating what you want, are far more positive and rewarding. Initially, when we start to ponder what we want to eat, outrageous requests may come to mind, or we sometimes still feel hungry after we have just eaten. It is very helpful to take a few moments and question ourselves to make sure that we are earnestly considering what we want to eat. Ask yourself whether you are hungry or if you just want to eat because you are bored.

There is a distinct difference between our desires to eat which are triggered from internal sensations of hunger and craving, and a desire to eat triggered because we have nothing better to do. Take time and focus on how you are feeling and try and describe how you feel. Give a name to what you are experiencing. Are you feeling hungry, thirsty, tired, angry, fed up, lonely, or some other feeling? By recognizing what you are feeling, you will not make the mistake of eating when you are not hungry, and you will be in a much better position to constructively deal with your situation.

If you are feeling hungry, focus on the foods that you urgently feel a craving for. Visualize the food that you want to eat, recall the taste of various foods that you might want. Choose the foods that you have the strongest urges and cravings for. You will be surprised at how well you can choose the foods that your body requires. You will soon recognize that you are meeting your dietary needs and eating what your body wants, because *the taste of the foods you eat becomes extremely delicious and you will experience an uplifting, happy feeling as you eat.*

When you first try to eat innately, you may still be unable to clue in to what you want to eat, and whatever you eat may not satisfy you. Sometimes we are not hungry but rather thirsty, so try drinking a glass of water. You will achieve best results in deciding what you want to eat if you are slightly hungry. However, you should not allow yourself to become overly hungry because when nutritive stores become depleted, and when there are too many shortages and your blood sugar is low, you will be compelled to eat without discrimination.

Many sweet lovers might initially say, "I feel hungry for a doughnut. Perhaps they do need to eat a doughnut, if they have accustomed themselves to satisfy their hunger with doughnuts. People who crave doughnuts should eat doughnuts. *If they do not eat that for which they have craved, they will eat everything else, and still turn around and eat the doughnut.* However, they should think about why they felt the need for the doughnut. They should reflect upon how they felt before eating the doughnut, how they have felt after eating the doughnut, and how they may get out of the cycle of needing to eat doughnuts, by finding an alternative steady supply of glucose so they may not crave for doughnuts. They should consider eating whole grain cereal for breakfast for a few mornings and see how they feel. The idea is to condition the body to develop a taste for slow-release carbohydrates in order to provide a steady supply of blood glucose without triggering the body's mechanisms to release insulin.

People who crave for sweets should also consider developing their muscles and cardiovascular system, so that muscles switch from burning glucose to burning fat. Once they develop a taste for whole grain food, their desire for sweets will subside. They will soon begin to realize that their mid-morning craving for a muffin or a doughnut disappears. If they still feel a need to eat a doughnut they should eat the doughnut without feeling guilty about it.

We tend to eat what we train ourselves to eat. For example, if we train ourselves to eat blobs of butter on our vegetables and loads of mayonnaise in our egg salad sandwiches, we will develop a taste for that. Then every time our bodies call for nutrients found in eggs or vegetables we will crave for the taste of these foods in the fashion that they were introduced to us, with butter or mayonnaise. To teach ourselves healthy eating habits we should develop a taste for vegetables without blobs of butter and sandwiches without loads of mayonnaise. We can use our *academic knowledge* while shopping to select and choose foods that are healthy for us, and during eating we can *innately learn* the tastes so we may crave for these foods when our bodies need them. Once we learn to satisfy our hunger by eating wholesome foods, we will start to crave wholesome foods.

It was mentioned in Chapter 12 that we are born with innate mechanisms that allow us to crave for foods according to the foods we need. Our cravings are based on our previous experiences with the foods that we eat. Therefore, it is important that we develop a taste for foods that are high in vitamins and minerals, contain a good source of slow release carbohydrates, and complete proteins. By eating these foods, we will develop our innate knowledge of these foods and we will develop a taste for them, and we will crave for them when their nutrients become needed in our bodies.

It is important that we subject our sensory eating mechanisms to a variety of different kinds of foods so we may learn their different characteristics - their tastes, textures, smells, colours, sounds, and how they make us feel after we have eaten them - so that we may have a large base of food items to choose from. When we expand our experience with food, it is as if our sensory vocabulary increases and it becomes easier for us to recognize the innate signals that will lead us to seek the nutrients we need.

It is wise to teach ourselves about the foods that become available to us at different times of the year. Foods that are in season are fresher and cheaper than those that are not. The changing seasons also cue us in to eating certain foods that our bodies require. For example, in the winter we need to eat foods that will give us more energy because we require more heat to keep ourselves warm. When snow falls and there is a fire burning in the fireplace, we may start to crave roasted chestnuts. While sitting outside in the shade of a tree in the summer we often crave for a slice of melon. Our energy needs and nutritional requirements change according to the seasonal conditions.

It is also a good idea to teach ourselves to eat the kinds of foods found in the regions that we live in, for it appears that each part of the world provides the ideal food source for its inhabitants. We humans must consider ourselves part of the land where we live, and recognize that we can be sustained by it. For instance, the people of the Arctic do very well on the foods their environment can provide for them. Although they do not have much milk, fresh fruits or vegetables in their diet, which consists mainly of seal or whale blubber and meat, few people are overweight and most people have strong teeth. By the same token, the diet of the people living in the mountains of Tibet consists of goat's milk, and seeds and plants that have been gathered from the land. People there still remain healthy and fit and are well known for longevity.

As we develop a taste for wholesome foods we will begin to gradually lose the taste for sugar and sweet tasting foods, and snacking between meals will subside. It is easy to develop a taste for whole grain foods because of the rewards we receive from the post-ingestional conditioning we experience by eating these foods. Our bodies quickly learn the calm contented feelings we experience after eating whole grain foods. This satisfaction results from the constant blood sugar levels that these foods can provide. We can change our eating habits by simply developing a taste for whole grain foods. By so doing we will get off the emotional rollercoaster we ride on when we eat sugar and sweets.

We also must reflect on how we are feeling during eating to appreciate and relish the foods we are eating and most importantly *to key in to the feelings of satiation and stop eating when we feel full.* Many people tend to eat what is placed in front of them, just because it is there. Perhaps they were taught to clean up their plates when they were young. Whatever the reason may be, if we eat after we feel full, we ignore the signals of satiation. Remember that there are two clusters of cells in the hypothalamus (Chapter 3) which are known as the satiation centers. When we eat all the nutrients that our bodies need, these centers will signal to us that we are full. If we do not use our satiation centers and continue to eat, we will deprive ourselves from the content feelings our satiation centers convey to us. When we cannot recognize the pleasure of being satiated, we will not learn to respond and know when we are feeling satiated. The body's "use it or lose it" rule also applies here. These centers will not develop to their potential and we will not stop eating when our nutritional requirements have been met. Many obese people take their cues and stop eating when they feel the discomfort of a distended stomach, eating far much more than they need and cannot recognize the point at which their nutritional needs have been met.

These centers are gaining a lot of attention lately. The pharmaceutical industry is now looking for chemical substances that will simulate the neurochemicals released from these centers, in an attempt to help obese people to feel satiated sooner. There is no need for this artificial external control. "Practice makes perfect." Once we start recognizing and responding to our satiation signals, and stop eating when full, our satiety centers will begin to produce all the appropriate neurochemicals that we need, and we will enjoy responding to our own sensations of contentment and satiation.

Developing our responsiveness to our sensory machinery does not happen overnight, nor will we lose "sixteen pounds in two weeks". We will become healthy, and will feel and look good as we start becoming aware of our sensations and feelings. When we learn to cue in to our various sensations of hunger, craving, and satiation, we will notice that our eating habits change, and gradually we will realize that fat layers are disappearing and we feel energetic, lively, and exhilarated, despite eating whatever we choose to eat. We will truly enjoy ourselves.

Chapter 22

Questions You Might Ask

Questions You Might Ask

It might seem an outrageous and a scary idea to seek our nutritional needs by examining the way we feel. **How can we trust that we will know what we want to eat? Should we not listen to the so-called "experts"? How can we be certain that our dietary requirements can be met by responding to our sensations and feelings of hunger and craving? Many illnesses and diseases are caused by malnutrition. How can someone in their right mind leave all the knowledge they have learned about nutrition and food, about recommended daily requirements of nutrients, calories, fat and protein content of food, and depend on their innate requests to provide them with proper nutrition?** These are questions that many readers are asking themselves.

Innate eating practices might appear alien to us, especially when we have been practising academic eating for most of our lives. But we must trust that innate eating is in our very nature.

Relating to food in terms of taste, texture, and how it satisfies our hunger is the way our bodies have always innately related to our food. But we have con-

stantly undermined this ability by consciously counting calories and rationing our food. To relate to our
food in the same way our bodies relate to food, does
not mean that we have to put out of commission all
academic knowledge we have learned about food. On
the contrary, our academic knowledge about food is a
profound and useful tool which we should use to gather
our food. When it comes to eating, we will do better if
we relate to the food in the same terms that our bodies
do, which is according to taste, texture, smell, how it
can satisfy our hunger, and how much we will enjoy
eating it.

When we want something to eat, we will eventually
have it, despite deliberation, resistance, and feelings of
guilt. This tells us that we cannot restrict our desires
and cravings and go against our nature. Not because
we are selfish, uncontrollable boors and slobs, but because our survival and well-being is at stake. Perhaps
the desire to eat is physical, or perhaps emotional.
Whatever it might be, *it is signaling to us to do something
to maintain our existence.* We must not ignore it.

To become an innate eater is to respond to all internal signals that our feelings relay to us. To be an innate
eater is to respond to our inner needs and to be attuned to our bodies.

If we cannot trust ourselves and want to be sure
that we meet all the recommended daily requirements
that we should eat, we can buy our food according to
our knowledge about its nutritional content. When we
go shopping for food, we can calculate all the caloric
values, and all the vitamin, mineral, carbohydrate, protein, and fat contents of the foods we buy. We can ex-

amine the freshness of what we purchase. We can ensure that food is clean and free of pesticides. We are paying for the food, so we must be sure of what we buy and bring home. We must make sure that our hard earned money does not buy us junk. We should not allow any junk foods to enter our house or even to pass the front gate! Junk food is any food containing only calories from sugar and fat, and very little, if any vitamins, minerals, or proteins. Sometimes we feel uncontrollable desires to eat junk, because junk foods contain sugar in large quantities, and we tend to become caught in a catch-22 sugar cycle (see Chapter 19).

Before going shopping for groceries, we should list what food items we need. Include all the varieties of proteins, lots of fresh fruits and vegetables, whole grain breads and cereals. If there are children in the house let the children voice what they want to eat. Have a bulletin board for food requests. Each member of the family can place their requests on the bulletin board. Be sure to buy every reasonable request on the board. Children sometimes just try their parents and request foods that they know their parents do not want them to have. Once they realize that their parents are prepared to comply with their request, they give up trying to make unreasonable requests for junk foods.

Studies examining food preferences have been done on children at the ages of six and seven. Children were allowed to do their own shopping and fill their grocery carts. The first few shopping sprees, children bought all kinds of junk. They stored the junk in a special cupboard assigned for their own use. They kept the junk in the cupboard and ate all other nutritious foods that they also had bought. Most children request things just to have them, or maybe because their friends have them. Once they have something they do not always really want it.

Often we notice this with Halloween candies. Children come home with all sorts of candies and junk foods. They open their loot bags and check every candy and chocolate bar that they have collected from the neighborhood. They even know which house gave them what. Then they pack up the goodies and put them away. Perhaps not all children will behave this way, but children who have developed or never lost innate eating responses hardly eat the candies they collect during trick-or-treat. Many mothers are surprised to find Halloween candies when cleaning closets in the new year. One mother has told me her little girl was saving the candies to give out for trick-or-treat next year. The child wanted to save money!

Telling children to refrain from sweets is not the answer to stop them from wanting to eat junk. The answer to the problem of getting children to eat healthy foods is to help them develop a taste for wholesome foods. Avoid training children to associate rewards with sweets or food in general to prevent eating from becoming a crutch for emotional stress. Allow them to receive their endorphins from playing, running, jumping, and racing the wind.

Always make available to children that other choice, wholesome foods like hot cereals for breakfast sprinkled with cinnamon and sweetened with a little honey. Fill lunch boxes with whole grain bread and peanut butter and banana, or any other filling they may request. Use skim milk, fresh fruit and juice. Make them a wholesome soup with barley and vegetables for when they come home from school. Prepare a modest but wholesome supper, of meat, potatoes, and lots and lots of vegetables. Give them carrot sticks, celery sticks, and cheese for snacks. Children will ask you to put some carrot sticks into their lunch box too. They will always choose the most nourishing and wholesome dinner, as long as parents do not make a big fuss over the chocolate bar that they might occasionally bring home just to tease their parents. Offer them an occasional home baked cookie made with whole grains. People do not have to refrain from the taste of sweet, but rather every time they eat sweet they should also eat slow release carbohydrates as well. This way our bodies will also have a chance to allow muscles to burn fat after utilizing the sugars we have eaten.

To ensure that we are meeting all the recommended daily requirements, we can practice *shopping academically* and *eating innately*. Allow individual meals and individual choices to develop out of innate requests. By ensuring that the academically purchased foods for the week are consumed within the week, we can be sure that recommended nutritional requirements are met on a weekly basis.

By developing a taste for slow-release carbohydrate meals and becoming attuned to our innate requests, we can take on a whole new attitude to eating. Our taste for sugars and other sweet desserts diminishes. When we provide a steady supply of energy to the brain, we can stay satiated for much longer periods of time. When our nutritional needs are met, requests for junk foods disappear.

Do not attempt to sweeten food. Allow yourself and your children to learn the natural tastes of wholesome foods without the taste of sugar. If children do not develop a taste for sweets as young babies, they will not crave them when they become older. Remember, eating habits are learned from experiences. The good news is that we can unlearn all our poor eating habits and replace them with good ones. We can train our bodies and minds to maximize all our capabilities, and focus on receiving joy and contentment from eating, rather than counting calories.

Many readers will be afraid of gaining weight when they stop calculating the caloric values of the foods they eat, and start to respond to innate requests.

We have always experienced innate eating requests in the form of cravings, but we have learned to suppress them. Every now and then, when we let our guard down we find ourselves reaching to eat the things we like, and then feel guilty and cut our rations even further, fearing we might gain weight. When we start to respond and eat the foods we are craving, we will enjoy ourselves more, experience more satisfaction from eating, our metabolic rate will rise, and we will burn more calories. The psychological benefits will also tip in our favor, we will feel more in control, and confident.

If you are concerned about gaining weight when eating what you crave, you can always increase your activities and begin to exercise regularly if you are not already doing so. As you develop your muscles and cardiovascular system, and as your nutritive reserves are replenished, you will find out that you are quite selective in what you eat without having to count calories and be concerned about the nutritional content of your meals.

Many readers are probably wondering how they would know if their cravings are triggered by shortages of specific nutrients or if their desire to eat is emotional?

Many people tend to reach for food or a cigarette or some other habit which automatically releases the neurochemicals they need to pacify their hurt. They use food to satisfy a stressful feeling that they are not even aware they have, nor do they realize that they are eating because they are feeling stressed out or hurt. By taking time and identifying what we feel, whether we feel hungry or hurt, and analyzing our emotional state before reaching out for food, we will be in a better position to recognize whether our hunger is brought about by an emotion or triggered by shortages of nutrients in our bodies.

We can start thinking of how we feel about ourselves, and identify the feeling we are experiencing, by giving the feeling a proper name. Take the time to reflect on how you feel and try to describe your feeling, whether you are feeling frustrated, angry, sad, or afraid, or something else. By defining what we feel, we can help ourselves to better understand why we are feeling that way. We will be in a better position to find solutions to our problems much more constructively than by resorting to eating to pacify ourselves.

We cannot become innate eaters overnight, the process is gradual. As we learn to respond to our sensations of hunger and cravings and maintain a steady blood sugar level by eating slow-release carbohydrates, we will gradually feel more energetic and more able to deal with our problems effectively and constructively.

It is important that we allow our children to grow up without clouding and cluttering their innate eating abilities. We can achieve this by trusting them when they tell us that they are not hungry, and not forcing them to eat foods they do not feel like eating. We do not have to be afraid that they will not be able to receive their proper nutrition if they do not eat what we think they should eat. They instinctively know what their little bodies need. We have no right to rob from them their ability to seek the foods they require. We can develop their abilities by asking them to taste new foods and describe their taste and texture and how it feels in their mouth. Help them to learn the tastes of various foods and allow them to eat what they want. Refrain from praising them for eating their food, nor do we need to bribe them to clean up their plates. Ensure that their experience with foods is a pleasant one, with no confrontations, arguments or distractions. Children, and all of us for that matter, need to learn and remember experiences with foods, and in everything else we encounter in our everyday living. These experiences ought to be as pleasant and fulfilling as possible. Our experience with food is an important component of how our body will relate to and select foods later.

Some readers might ask what about fat? Would it not be better for our health to avoid eating foods with higher fat content?

We crave fatty foods because we have trained ourselves to add fat to the other foods that are rich in vitamins, proteins, and of course sweet desserts. We do not necessarily crave for fat itself. For example, if we train ourselves to find our iodine from eating fried fish instead of poached fish, or from eating iodized salt richly sprinkled on french fries or salted potato chips, then every time there is a shortage of iodine in our body we will crave french fries with salt, salted chips, or fried fish, instead of poached fish or boiled potatoes with salt.

Our bodies need a large variety of nutrients, minerals, vitamins, and proteins that are found in various foods, most of which also contain molecules of fat and carbohydrates. We might even crave for fatty foods whenever fat soluble vitamins are needed by our cells, or when our blood sugar level is low. If we start artificially loading our food with fat and sugar, we will take in more energy than our bodies require, and this can pose major problems to our energy balancing mechanisms. We must develop good eating habits and learn the taste of food without added sugars and fats. We must learn to satisfy our hunger and cravings with natural, unprocessed foods that are rich in vitamins, minerals, proteins and slow-release carbohydrates, without loading these foods with the extra calories and accompanying ill-effects of fat and/or sugar. We can do this by staying away from processed foods. We can shop wisely and avoid purchasing foods loaded with added fat and sugars.

The metabolic functions of our bodies are innately controlled, and we have innate abilities to seek and select the specific nutrients required at the cellular level.

By using our innate abilities to select our foods we will meet our nutritional needs. Our sensory mechanisms are designed to release neurochemicals and endorphins to alert us to our needs, and when we satisfy our needs, we are rewarded with pleasant uplifting feelings of happiness and joy. In enjoying what we do, we will learn to recognize what we must do to become healthy, happy, and fit.

Rejoice! We are BORN TO BE FIT.

Glossary

A

Acetone: A volatile chemical compound CH_3COOH_3 It is an organic compound used in paint thinner and nail polish remover.

Acetylcholine: One of the first neurotransmitters discovered, found in the brain and spinal cord ganglia of the autonomic nervous system.

Agonist: A facilitator. An a agonistic drug facilitates the effect of a particular neurotransmitter.

Anorexia nervosa: A disorder that most frequently afflicts young women. They become overly concerned with their weight and starve themselves, sometimes to the point of death.

Anabolism: The process in living organisms by which nutrients are changed into living tissue, constructive metabolism.

Assimilation: The action of the body that changes digested foods and other materials into body tissue.

Autonomic nervous system: The portion of the nervous system that controls vegetative functions of the body. It consists of two divisions. The sympathetic division mediates functions that accompany arousal. The parasympathetic division mediates functions that occur during a relaxed state.

B

Brain stem: An important part of the brain from the medulla to the midbrain.

Bulimia: An eating disorder associated with self-induced vomiting after gorging or binge eating.

C

Calorie: The amount of heat needed to raise the temperature of one cubic centimeter of water one degree centigrade.

Catabolism: The process of changing body tissue into waste products and Destructive metabolism.

Conditioned emotional response: A conditioned response occurring when a neutral stimulus is followed by an aversive stimulus, causing the secretion of stress related hormones.

Cerebral cortex: The layer of gray matter forming the outer shell of the cerebral hemispheres of the brain. It is highly developed in mammals.

Cortical areas: Distinct zones of the cortex characterized by their cellular architecture and function.

Catecholamine: A class of neurotransmitters that includes dopamine.

Carboxyl group: COHO group.

CSF: Cerebrospinal fluid.

D

Dendrites: Multiple branches of a neuron that receive numerous synaptic contacts form axon terminals thus collecting signals and transmitting them to the cell body.

Digestion: The process of changing food in the mouth, the stomach, and the intestine by the chewing, and actions of intestinal juices, enzymes, and bacteria so that it can be absorbed by the body.

Dopamine: A catecholamine neurotransmitter that is implicated in relieving pain and relaxation.

E

Emotion: Psychical excitement, associated with love, hate, rage, fear, happiness, sadness, etc.

Endocrine system: A group of glands in various parts of the body which release hormones directly into the bloodstream, to initiate or suppress the action of other body organs or cells.

Endogenous peptides: A class of proteins produced by the brain or the pituitary cells that act as opiates, including endorphins and enkephalins.

Enkephalin: A peptide neurotransmitter that acts like morphine.

Glossary

F

Fatty acid: A by-product of the metabolism of fat, the other by-product being glycerol.

Fructose: The sweetest tasting of all sugars which has the same chemical formula as glucose but a different molecular structure. Fructose is the sugar found in fruits.

G

Glucose: A simple sugar molecule. Not as sweet tasting as sucrose (table sugar)

Glucagon: A pancreatic hormone that triggers the liver cells to convert glycogen into glucose.

Glycogen: An animal polysaccharide that is stored in the liver and converted to blood glucose.

Glycerol: A triglyceride alcohol converted into glucose by the liver. Fat is composed of fatty acids and glycerol.

H

Hormones: Chemical substances secreted by the endocrine glands.

Hypoactive: Not working at full capacity.

Hypoglycemia: A physiological state characterized by a low level of blood glucose.

Hyperglycemia: A physiological state characterized by high levels of blood glucose.

Hypothalamus: A cluster of neurons on the forebrain beneath the thalamus. Despite its small size, it plays an important role in vital functions, including feeding, drinking, sexual behavior, sleep, temperature regulation, emotion, and hormone balance.

Histofluorescence technique: A technique that exposes brain tissue to formaldehyde gas causing noradrenergic neurons to fluorescence a bright yellow under ultraviolet light.

I

Islet Of Langerhans: Numerous clusters of endocrine glands in the pancreas that produce insulin.

Immune system: The system body uses to protects itself from foreign invasions of bacteria, viruses, or disease by producing antibodies.

Insulin: A pancreatic hormone that allows the entry of glucose into the cells, assists the conversion of glucose into glycogen, and transports fat cells to fat tissue deposits.

K

Ketone bodies: Organic acid produced in the body from the breakdown of fats, which can be utilized by the brain for energy.

L

Limbic system: A group of brain regions at the base of the brain, including the anterior thalamic nuclei, amygdala, hippocampus, limbic cortex, and the hypothalamus and interconnecting fiber bundles.

Lactose: The principal sugar in milk.

M

Membrane: A thin sheet or layer serving as a covering or lining, as for an organ or tissue.

Metabolism: The sum of all the physical and chemical changes that take place in an organism including all chemical reactions and the liberation of energy.

Mitochondrion: The cell organelle in which the chemical reaction of the Krebs cycle takes place.

N

Naloxone: A drug that blocks opiate receptors and the effects of endogenous and exogenous opiates. Used in treating overdoses of opium and its derivatives.

Neuron: The nerve cell. It consists of a cell body, containing the nucleus, and outgrowths of dendrites, and a single axon.

Neurotransmitter: A chemical substance involved in the transmission of the nerve signal at a chemical synapse. There are probably dozens of such transmitters on the brain.

Glossary

P

Phagocytosis: The action of special cells engulfing foreign bodies and debris caused by cellular degeneration. The cells that perform this function are called phagocytes.

Pheromones: Chemicals released by one animal that affect the behavior or physiology of another animal.

Pituitary Gland: The master endocrine gland situated at the base of the brain. It is composed of two parts. The anterior pituitary releases hormones in response to the hypothalamic hormones. The posterior pituitary produces oxytocin or antidiuretic hormones in response to stimulations from its neuronal cells.

Peristalsis: The rhythmic wave-like motion of the walls of the elementary canal and certain other hollow organs like the intestines. Alternate muscular contractions and dilatations move the contents of the tube onward.

R

Retina: The light-sensitive neuronal tissue which lines the inner surface of the back of the eyeball.

S

Satiety: Cessation of hunger produced by the adequate supply of nutrients in the body.

Species-typical behavior: Behavior that is typical of most members of a given species. Generally the term refers to a behavior that does not appear to have to be learned.

T

Target cell: A type of cell that is directly affected by a hormone or a nerve fiber.

T-cell: A white blood cell which arises from the thalamus gland and regulates the immune system by fighting off infection.

References

Abel, E.L., and Sokol, R.J. Fetal alcohol syndrome is now a leading cause of mental retardation. *Lancet, 1986, 22,122.*

Aschoff, J. et al., "Meal Timing in Humans during Isolation without Time Cues". Journal of Biological Rhythms 1, no 2 (1986): 160; in Martin C. Moore-Ede and Charles A. Czeisler, eds., *Mathematical Model of Circadian Sleep-Wake Cycle,* (New York: Raven Press, 1948, 209).

Beecher, H.K. *Measurement of Subjective Responses: Quantitative Effects of Drugs.* New York: Oxford University Press, 1959.

Bennett, G. *Eating Matters,* 1988 Heinemann Kingswood: London.

Birch, L.L. Marlin, D.W. 1982 I don't like it; I never tried it : Effects of exposure on two-year-old children's food preferences. *Appetite, 353-360.*

Birch, L.L., McPhee, L., Shoba, B.C., Steinberg, L., and Krehbiel, R. "Clean up your plate": Effects of child feeding practices on the conditioning of meal size. *Learning and Motivation, 1987, 18,301-317.*

Brala, P.M., and Hagen, R.L. Effects of sweetness perception and calorie value of a preload on short term intake. *Physiology and Behavior, 1983, 30,1-9.*

Breisch, S.T., Zelman, F.P., and Hoebel, B.G., Hyperphagia and obesity following serotonin depletion by intraventricular p-chlorphenylalane. *Science, 1976, 192,382-384.*

Brownell K.D., Greenwood M.R.C., Stellar E., and Shreger, E.E., The effects of repeated cycles of weight loss and regain in rats. *Physiology and Behavior. 1986, 38, 459- 464.*

Burton, M.J., Rolls, E.T., and Mora, F. Effects of hunger on responses of neurons in the lateral hypothalaumus to the sight and taste of food. *Experimental Neurology, 1976, 51, 668-677.*

Cannon, W. B. *The Wisdom of The Body* (2nd ed.) 1939, New York : Norton.

Carlson, N.L., *Physiology of Behavior.* Boston: Allyn and Bacon, 1991, p 528.

References

Carlson, N.L., Physiology *of Behavior*. Boston: Allyn and Bacon, 1991, P. 64

Carlson, N.L., *Physiology of Behavior*. Boston: Allyn and Bacon, 1991, p 437.

Carney, R.M. and Goldberg, A.P. Weight gain after cessation of cigarette smoking: A possible role for adipose-tissue lipoprotein lipase. *New England Journal of Medicine, 310,* 1984: 614-616

Changeux, Jean-Pierre. Translated from *L'Homme Neuronial,* Librairie Artheme Fayard 1983. As quoted by Dr. Laurence Garey. *The Neuronial Man, 1985, 113.* Pantheon Books, New York.

Chang, F.L.F., and Greenough, W.T. Lateralized effects of monocular training on dendritic branching in adult split-brain rats. *Brain Research, 1982, 232, 283-292.*

Costill, D.L, Dalsky, G.P., Fink, W.J., Effects of caffeine ingestion on metabolism and exercise performance. *Medicine and Science in Sports, 10, 1978: 1155-158*

Davis, M.C. Self-selection of diet by newly weaned infants. *American Journal of Disease of Children, 1928, 36,651-679.*

Damsma, G., Day, and Fibiger, H.C. Lack of tolerance to nicotine-induced dopamine release in nucleus accumbens. *European Journal of Pharmacology, 1989, 168, 363-365.*

De Angelis *Real Moments 1984* Delcorte Press N.Y.

Jean Jacques d'Ortous de Mairan, translated from *Histoire Del'Acadamie Royale des Sciences, (Paris* 1729) as quoted in Alexander Borbely, *Secrets of Sleep,* 1968. New York: Basic Books.

Freud Sigmund , Introductory Lectures on Psychoanalysis. English translation by James Strachey. Penguin Books, P, 402 First published in *The Standard Edition of the Complete Psychological Works of Sigmund Freud.* By the Hogarth Press: London 1963.

Fomon, S.J. Factors influencing food consumption in the human infant. *International Journal of Obesity,* 1980, 4,348-350.

Gessa, G.L., Muntoni, F., Collu, M., Vargiu, L., and Mereu, G. Low doses of ethanol activates dopaminergic neurons in the ventral tegmental area. *Brain Research 1985, 348, 201-204.*

Greenough, W.T., and Volkmar, F.R. Patterns of dendritic branching in occipital cortex of rats reared in complex environments. *Experimental Neurology*, 1973, 40,491-504.

Harris, R.B.S., Bruch, R.C., and Martin, R.J. In vitro evidence for an inhibitor of lipogenesis in serum from overfed obese rats. *American Journal of Physiology*, 1989, 257,R326-R336.

Himmi, T., Boyer, A., and Orsini, J.C. Changes in lateral hypothalamic neuronal activity accompanying hyper-and hypoglycemia. *Physiology and Behavior*, 1988, 44,347-354.

Knoll, J. Satietin: A centrally acting potent anorectic substance with long-lasting effect in human and mammalian blood. *Polish Journal of Pharmacology and Pharmacy*, 1982, 34,3-16. As quoted in - Carlson, N.L., *Physiology of Behavior*. Boston: Allyn and Bacon, 1991

Kramer, F.M., Jeffery, R.W., Forster, J.L., and Snell, M.K. Long-term follow-up of behavioral treatment for obesity: Patterns of regain among men and women. *International Journal of Obesity*, 1989, 13,123-136.

LeBlanc, J., and Cabanac, M. Cephalic postprandial thermogenesis in human subjects. *Physiology and Behavior*, 1989, 46,479-482.

Leibowitz, S.F., and Weiss, G.F., Walsh, U.A., and Viswanath, D. Medial hypothalamic serotonin: Role in circadian patterns of feeding and macronutrient selection. *Brain Research*, 1989, 503,132-140.

Leonard T.K., Watson R.R., and Mohs M. E., the effects of caffeine on various body systems: A review, *Journal of The American Dietetic Association*, 87 1987:1048-1053.

Leonard, T. K., Watson, R.R. and Mohs M.E., Caffeine can increase brain serotonin levels, *Nutrition Today* 46 1988: 366-367

Loftus, E.F. Leading questions and eyewitness report. *Cognitive Psychology*, 1975, 7,560-572

Luria, A.R. *The Mind of a Mnemonist*, 1988. New York Basic Books.

Lyman, B. Nutritional value of food groups and characteristics of foods preferred during various emotions. *Journal of Psychology*, 1982, 112; 121-127.

References

Murphy, M.R. Bowie, D.L. & Pert, C.B. Copulation elevate plasma B-endorphin in the male hamster. *Soc. Neuroscience Abs.*, 1979 p. 470.

Newman, D. "Tidal and Lunar Rhythms" in Juergen Aschoff, ed., Biological Rhythms vol. 4 of *Handbook of Behavioral Neurobiology*, New York Plenum Press 1981, 372.

Olds J, Commentary. In *Brain Stimulation and Motivation*, edited by E.S. Valenstien. Glenview, Ill.:Scott, Foresman, 1973.

Rodin, L., Schank, D., Striegel-Moore, R. Psychological features of obesity. *Medical Clinics of North America, 1989, 73,* 47-66.

Rolls, E.T., Murzi, E., Yaxley, S., Thorpe, S.J., and Simpson S.J. Sensory-specific satiety: food specific reduction responsiveness of ventral fore-brain neurons after feeding in the monkey. *Brain Research, 1986,76, 135-164.*

Roper. S.D., *Science News* V. 136 Nov. 1989. Rick Weiss reports from Phoenix, Ariz. *At the annual meeting of the Society for Neuroscience*

Rosenzweig, M.A. Experience, memory, and the brain. *American Psychologist, 1984,39,365-376*

Rothwell, N.J. and Stock, M.J., A role for brown adipose tissue in diet-induced thermogenesis. *Nature, 1979,281,31-35*

Sato, M., Chen, C.C., Akiyama, K., and Otsuki, S. Acute exacerbation of paranoid psychotic state after long term abstinence in patients with previous methamphetamine psychosis *Biological Psychiatry, 1983, 18,429-440.*

Selye, H. *The Stress of Life*. McGraw Hill, 1958,186.

Sherwood, L. *Human Physiology,* 1991 West Publishing Company, St. Paul. 1990,607.

Slochower, J. and Kaplan, S.P. Anxiety, perceived control, and eating in obese and normal weight persons. *Appetite, 1980, 75-83.*

Stanly, B.G., Shwartz, D.H., Hernendaz, L., Leibowitz, S.F., and Hoebel, G.B. Patterns of extracellular 5-hydrooxyindoleacetic acid 5-(HIAA) In Paraventricular hypothalamus (PVN): Relation to circadian rhythm and deprivation induced eating behavior. *Pharmacology Biochemistry and Behavior, 1989, 33,257-360.*

Born to Be Fit

Steen, S.N., Oppliger, R.A., and Brownell, K.D. Metabolic effects of repeated weight loss or gain in adolescent wrestlers. *Journal of American Medical Association*, 1988, 47-50.

Sternbach, R.A. Pain: *A Psychological Analysis*. New York Academic Press, 1968.

Sulser, F., and Sanders-Bush, E. From Neurochemical to molecular pharmacology of antidepressants. In *Tribute to B.B. Brodie*, Edited by E, Costa. Raven Press, 1989, New York.

Tordoff, M.G. How do non nutritive sweeteners increase food intake? *Appetite*, 1988, 11,5-11.

Traskmann, L., Asberg, M. Bertilsson, L., and Sjostrand, L. Monamine metabolites in CSF and suicidal behavior. *Archives Of General Psychiatry*, 1981, 38,631-636.

Turner, A.M., and Greenough, W.T., Differential rearing effects on rats visual cortex synapsis. I. Synaptic and neuronal density and synapsis per neuron. *Brain Research*, 1985, 329,195-203.

Vogel, G.W., Neill, D., Hagler, M., and Kors, D. A New animal model of endogenous depression: A summary of present findings. *Neuroscience and Biobehavioral Reviews*, 1990, 14,85-92.

Wegscheidre Hyman ,J. "*The Light Book*" 1990, 9-10. Jeremy P. Thacher, Los Angeles

Welle, S.L., Nair, K.S., and Campbell, R.G. Failure of chronic B-adrenergic blockade to inhibit overfeeding-induced thermogenesis in humans. *American Journal of Physiology*, 1989, 256,R653-R658.

Whitney E, Hamilton, E.M., Rolfs, S. *Understanding Nutrition*, West Publishing Company, 1990, 407.

Wise, R.A. Psychomotor stimulant properties of addictive drugs. *Annals of New York Acdamy Of Sciences*, 1988, 537,228-234.

286